Titles previously published in
YOUR PERSONAL HEALTH SERIES

YOUR PERSONAL HEALTH SERIES

ASSOCIATION
MÉDICALE
CANADIENNE

CANADIAN
MEDICAL
ASSOCIATION

When a Child Has Diabetes

Third Edition

Denis Daneman, MB, BCh, FRCPC
Marcia Frank, RN, MHSc, CDE
Kusiel Perlman, MD, FRCPC

KEY PORTER BOOKS

Library and Archives Canada Cataloguing in Publication

Daneman, Denis
        When a child has diabetes / Denis Daneman, Marcia Frank, Kusiel Perlman—3rd ed.

ISBN 978-1-55470-255-8

        1. Diabetes in children—Popular works.
I. Frank, Marcia II. Perlman, Kusiel III. Title.

RJ420.D5D36 2010   618.92'462   C2009-905865-0

ONTARIO ARTS COUNCIL
CONSEIL DES ARTS DE L'ONTARIO

The publisher gratefully acknowledges the support of the Canada Council for the Arts and the Ontario Arts Council for its publishing program. We acknowledge the support of the Government of Ontario through the Ontario Media Development Corporation's Ontario Book Initiative.

We acknowledge the financial support of the Government of Canada through the Book Publishing Industry Development Program (BPIDP) for our publishing activities.

Key Porter Books Limited
Six Adelaide Street East, Tenth Floor
Toronto, Ontario
Canada M5C 1H6
www.keyporter.com

Diagrams: Lianne Friesen
Editor: Paula Chabanais
Electronic formatting: Heidy Lawrance Associates

Printed and bound in Canada
10 11 12 13 14 6 5 4 3 2 1

For those whose lives are touched by diabetes
and those with diabetes whose lives have touched us.

Do You Want to Raise Happier, Healthier Children?

So Do We!

Join the SickKids Family Knowledge Group
and be a part of the SickKids vision:
Healthier Children. A Better World. ™

At The Hospital for Sick Children (SickKids) we are experts in patient care, but we also make products that families can use in their everyday lives.

We are looking for empowered and excited parents to share opinions, ideas, and thoughts on how we can improve and develop better products.

Membership to this unique group is absolutely *free* and entitles you to receive timely and relevant information and practical tips on important child health topics—wonderful and important information to have and share with friends!

Members have the opportunity to participate in focus groups, book reviews (free books!), and mini surveys. If you don't have the time to engage in any of the activities...no problem! You will still have access to helpful tips sent to members, via email, on a regular basis

Signing up is quick and easy—please visit this website: www.skfamilyknowledgegroup.ca or call 416.813.7654 x2971.

Contents

Acknowledgments

We would like to acknowledge a number of individuals who have made direct and important contributions to this book: Margo Small, the social worker on our diabetes team at The Hospital for Sick Children, provided us with invaluable assistance in writing Chapters Seven and Eight, and Jennifer Buccino RD, MEd, CDE, a dietitian on our diabetes team, wrote Chapter Four for this edition. Janice Biehn provided initial writing and editorial support, for which we are grateful.

Other members of the diabetes team have given ongoing support, and have reviewed the content along the way to ensure accuracy and comprehensiveness. They include our diabetes nursing and dietitian colleagues: Ana Artiles-Sisk, RN, CDE; Janet Ruston, RN, CDE; Shaun Barrett, RN, BScN, CDE; Angela Stone, RN, BScN; Esther Assor, RD; and Vanita Pais, RD, CDE, as well as our fellow pediatric endocrinologists, Drs. Diane Wherrett, Étienne Sochett, Jill Hamilton, and Jacqueline Curtis. We all owe a large debt of gratitude to Dr. Robert Ehrlich, the originator of the interdisciplinary diabetes team at The Hospital for Sick Children, who encouraged and supported us from the time we started our careers in diabetes care.

Denis Daneman, MB, BCh, FRCPC
Marcia Frank, RN, MHSc, CDE
Kusiel Perlman, MD, FRCPC

Foreword

The discovery of insulin by Frederick Banting and Charles Best, at the University of Toronto in 1921, suddenly and dramatically changed the outlook for people with type 1 diabetes. No longer was it a fatal disease, and no longer did health care professionals need to watch helplessly as children succumbed. Now there was treatment. The Hospital for Sick Children in Toronto quickly made a commitment to the care of children and adolescents with diabetes, a tradition that continues today. One of the first physicians to become involved in both diabetes care and research was Dr. Laurie Chute, followed by such eminent clinicians as Dr. Harry Bain and Dr. Robert Ehrlich.

In the 1960s it became evident that diabetes care and education were too complex to be handled in the traditional medical model—that is, through occasional visits to the doctor by the child or teen and his or her family. Rather, what was needed was an interdisciplinary health care team consisting of physicians, nurses, dietitians, and behavioral specialists, all bringing their unique training and expertise to bear on the care of this complex condition. The diabetes team was the first of the interdisciplinary teams now standard in many areas of health care.

Since most diabetes care occurs in the home, at school, or elsewhere outside the hospital or doctor's office, it has also become apparent that the care of children and teens with diabetes requires a family-centered approach: both the child or teen and the family are intimately involved in decisions that affect not only the diabetes, but all aspects of their lives.

This book is intended primarily for those involved in the care of children and teens with diabetes: parents, other family members, teachers and other school personnel, sports coaches, camp counselors, and others, not forgetting the children and teens themselves. It is essential that those affected know as much as possible about the disorder. While we do not intend to present the last word on every subject, we hope you will find this a useful first step in learning about diabetes and its management, and a comforting reference when things seem not to be going quite according to plan.

Where does our information come from? We have all learned from our training, our mentors, our day-to-day work, and, most particularly, from the children, teens, and families whose experiences with diabetes constantly yield new information, new approaches, and new coping strategies.

There are a few important caveats to remember as you read this book. First, different diabetes health care teams have different approaches to some or all of the aspects of diabetes care we deal with here. If you are confused by something we have written, or it conflicts with the approach of your health care providers, discuss it with them. Most often you will find that what we have provided is a variation, rather than a radically different approach.

Secondly, this book was written in 1998, revised in 2002, and again in 2009—things change! We expect that biomedical research will continue to advance our understanding of many aspects of diabetes care in the foreseeable future. So expect an evolution in our thinking in years to come.

Finally, not everything works for everybody. If something doesn't seem applicable to you or your child, discuss it with your team. Once you have a good understanding of the condition, work with your team to do some further experimentation. Try things out and see how successful they are. If they work well, tell us about them—we're always ready to learn.

We present this work in the proud tradition of excellence in diabetes care, education, and research that has been the trademark of The Hospital for Sick Children for almost ninety years. If in some small way it lessens the burden of diabetes management for our readers, we will have fulfilled our mission.

Introduction

Heather is nine and she's a livewire. A tall, thin child with straight blonde hair and bangs, she's bright and bold and independent. Drama is her forte and she sings and travels with a children's opera chorus. For Heather, each new experience is an adventure; she refuses to let diabetes change her life.

Tommy is a charming, cherubic child of two and a half. He spends hours pretending he's a firefighter, gathering his siblings and playmates into fire-fighting squads. Tommy has diabetes and these days he would much rather "cook" in his play fire station than eat real food. His unpredictable eating makes it harder to manage his diabetes safely.

Sonia is in the tenth grade and a serious student. Although she's a quiet girl, she enjoys an active social life and has a lot of friends. Sonia and her family are amazingly resilient; not only have they mastered a new language and become integrated into a new culture in the past year and a half, they are also well on their way to mastering Sonia's newly diagnosed diabetes.

For each of these youngsters and their families, diabetes, and all that goes with it, is a challenge that they are forced to meet each and every day. With each milestone in life, a new aspect of living with diabetes is revealed. Indeed, the immediate and long-term health and emotional well-being of the child, and to some extent of the entire family, depend on the successful integration of diabetes into their lives.

What exactly is diabetes? What is involved in "managing" or "controlling" diabetes? How do growth and development affect diabetes and, conversely, how does diabetes impact on growth and development? This book addresses these and many other questions, so that friends and relatives, health care professionals, teachers, coaches, school bus drivers, and camp counselors can more effectively support children and their families as they embark on life's journey with diabetes.

The information and insights presented here will interest both those who are new to diabetes in young people and those who are experienced with it. Each phase of adapting to the disorder and each stage of child and family development brings new questions, concerns, and expectations related to diabetes management. Families and care providers will find this book an excellent resource, but it has its limitations. It cannot and should not replace the comprehensive education program provided to the child and family, at the time of diagnosis and beyond, by a team of experienced health care professionals.

Gathering together the collected wisdom of the pediatric diabetes team, including children, adolescents, and their families, this is a practical guide for young people with diabetes, their families, and everyone else who cares about them.

The Diabetes Team
To meet the complex and ever-changing demands of living with diabetes, all children, teens, and their families should have access to and be able to work with an experienced diabetes health care team. Each professional in this group brings unique experience and expertise to the care of the child or teen

and the support of the family. At the center of this interdisciplinary team, however, are the child and the family, because care must be tailored to meet their individual needs. The "core" team should also include:

- a physician, usually a pediatric endocrinologist or diabetologist
- a diabetes nurse (often called a diabetes nurse educator)
- a diabetes dietitian
- a social worker, psychologist, and/or other counselor such as a Child Life Specialist

Members of the "extended" team, in addition to other family members, include:

- the family practitioner or pediatrician
- school personnel
- recreation workers
- the pharmacist
- babysitters
- others who share responsibility for child care

What Do You Need to Learn and Why?

In the following chapters we will answer these important questions:

- What happens when someone develops diabetes?
- What is the difference between type 1 diabetes and type 2 diabetes?
- What does "blood glucose balance" mean and what affects it?
- What do we need to know about insulin?
- Why do we need a meal plan?
- How do we assess the effectiveness of diabetes care routines?

The diabetes team

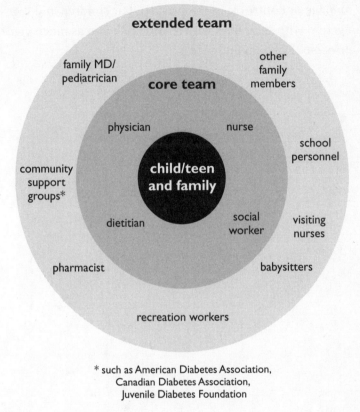

extended team

family MD/
pediatrician

core team

other
family
members

physician   nurse

child/teen
and family

school
personnel

community
support
groups*

dietitian   social
worker

visiting
nurses

pharmacist   babysitters

recreation workers

* such as American Diabetes Association,
Canadian Diabetes Association,
Juvenile Diabetes Foundation

- What do we do when blood glucose is out of balance?
- How do we deal with the emotional impact of diabetes?
- How does diabetes care differ at different ages?
- Do we need to worry about diabetes complications?
- Will the child become a healthy adult?
- What is the future of diabetes?

Diabetes at any age is a real challenge. It imposes itself on virtually all aspects of daily life. Learning about diabetes, and how to manage or control it, is essential so that children and teens can get on with their lives with as little risk and as much vigor as possible. Read on and learn.

ONE

Overview

It had been a hot and humid summer. Jim and Ruth didn't think it was terribly unusual that their eight-year-old son, Danny, seemed to be drinking so much water. They also felt that, since he was drinking so much, it was normal for him to get up a couple of times each night to urinate. What started to worry them was the weight loss: in June he had weighed 56 pounds (25 kg) at his annual check-up, and now, in mid-July, he looked skinny and weighed in at only 49 pounds (22 kg). The neighbors said not to worry—it was summer, and Danny was burning up so much energy at day camp that the weight loss was just part of his normal development.

Ruth's concern reached a crisis point when Danny started to feel listless and vomited three times one Sunday morning. Jim was out of town on business, so it was Ruth's decision to head to the hospital to see what was going on.

The doctors and nurses in the emergency room seemed to pick up the clues right away: the increased urination and thirst, coupled with weight loss, and now vomiting and dehydration, all pointed to diabetes. They confirmed their suspicions with a quick urine check and blood tests; both showed high amounts of glucose. Danny was admitted and immediately given an intravenous drip to replace fluids, and the hormone insulin, which would help deal with the excess glucose. Within hours, he began to look more like his former self and was feeling much better. By the next morning he was well enough to be taken off the intravenous and receive his first insulin injection before breakfast. His father returned quickly from his business trip. It was time for the family to begin to learn the ropes of living with diabetes.

What Is Diabetes?

To a child with diabetes, the very first syllable of the word can seem frightening. Younger children think in very concrete terms, and many wonder if a person with "di"abetes is going to die. But the word "diabetes" comes from the Greek word for "to run through" or "to siphon." Diabetes has been known since about 1500 B.C., when the first medical document referring to excessive urine production was written. Sometime between 30 B.C. and A.D. 45, Aretaeus of Cappadocia, a Greek physician, applied the term to people who had to urinate frequently. When doctors in the seventeenth century further discovered that the urine was sweet, they added the Latin word mellitus, meaning honey. In fact, an early method of diagnosis was to pour the urine on the ground; if ants scurried to the site, the doctor's suspicion was confirmed.

People excrete glucose in their urine when they are missing the essential hormone insulin. A hormone is a chemical "messenger" that travels from one part of the body to tell another part what to do. Only with the help of insulin can the body's metabolic processes release the energy from the glucose in the food we eat, to let our muscles work, to produce our body heat, and for the continual growth, renewal, and repair of the billions of cells that make up our bodies. (Metabolic processes are the complex series of chemical reactions that work to either produce or employ energy for the functioning of the body.) Without insulin, we can't survive.

The digestive system

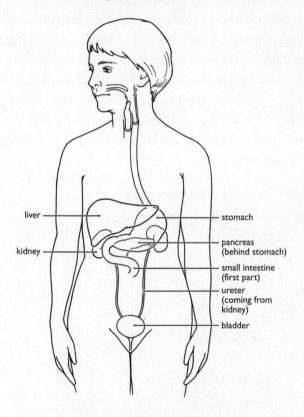

liver

kidney

stomach

pancreas
(behind stomach)

small intestine
(first part)

ureter
(coming from
kidney)

bladder

Insulin is made in the pancreas (an organ located just behind the stomach) by highly specialized cells known as beta cells. These are found within the pancreas, in islands of tissue named the islets of Langerhans, for the scientist, Paul Langerhans, who discovered them.

In children and teens with diabetes, the majority of the beta cells have been destroyed. This means that little or no insulin can be produced. The only way they can once again use glucose for energy is to replace the missing insulin. At present this can only be done effectively by daily insulin injections or by continuously infusing insulin under the skin by means of a pump. When children develop diabetes, only the insulin-producing cells are destroyed. The rest of the pancreas is healthy and continues to produce digestive enzymes and another hormone called glucagon.

Type 1 diabetes is characterized by the absolute or relative inability to produce insulin. Most people with diabetes are adults and have type 2 diabetes, which means that they can produce some insulin but it doesn't work properly to use up all the available glucose.

The pancreas

beta cell
(produces insulin)

alpha cell
(produces glucagon)

islet of Langerhans

other pancreatic tissues
(produces
digestive juices)

microscopic view of pancreas cells

Types of Diabetes

Most people know somebody with diabetes. Friends and colleagues are quick to offer well-meaning advice about their 50-year-old uncle who was recently diagnosed with diabetes, or their sister who had diabetes while she was pregnant. They tell stories of people who had to cut out sweets and trim fat from their diets, take medication and exercise, but didn't require daily insulin injections. Then why do most children with diabetes require insulin injections?

The simple answer is that most children develop a different type of diabetes than most adults. Children with diabetes generally have type 1—previously known as insulin-dependent diabetes mellitus (IDDM), or juvenile diabetes. In type 1 diabetes, the pancreas loses its ability to produce any or enough insulin. By the time the symptoms of the disorder have developed, at least 80 percent of the beta cells have already been destroyed. Nobody knows for certain how long this destruction progresses before diagnosis, but it is probably many months or years. Type 1 diabetes is usually diagnosed before age 40, and most commonly in children aged 2 to 16. Of all the people with diabetes in North America, type 1 affects only 10 percent. Of that 10 percent, half are under the age of 20.

The rest of the diabetes population has type 2 diabetes, formerly known as non-insulin-dependent diabetes mellitus (NIDDM). The beta cells are still present in the pancreas, but they don't make enough insulin, and/or the insulin they produce doesn't work well enough to keep blood glucose levels normal. This occurs most often in overweight adults, but more and more younger people are being diagnosed with type 2 diabetes, most likely because of the rising rate of obesity among children and teens. The first line of treatment is strict dietary management, with a focus on healthy eating and a goal of achieving and maintaining a healthy weight. Those with type 2 diabetes are also advised and encouraged to quit smoking and to become more active by reducing their sedentary activities, such as watching television. In addition to these strategies, an oral medication is sometimes used to help the pancreas make more insulin or to make the insulin work better. Sometimes the doctor will also prescribe insulin injections for people with type 2 diabetes, but this doesn't change the diagnosis to type 1.

Some women develop diabetes during pregnancy. This is known as gestational diabetes. Women with gestational diabetes need the help of an expert team to achieve excellent blood glucose control, to give them the best possible chance of having a healthy baby. Treatment involves careful monitoring, some

Types of Diabetes

	Type 1	Type 2
also called	insulin-dependent diabetes mellitus (IDDM) juvenile diabetes childhood diabetes	non-insulin-dependent diabetes mellitus (NIDDM) maturity-onset diabetes adult-onset diabetes
usually diagnosed in	younger people (between infancy and 40)	older people (over 40; incidence increases with age); often people with a significant weight problem
insulin is	eventually totally absent	produced, but too little or too ineffective to deal with the demands of the body
accounts for	about 10% of all people with diabetes	90% of all people with diabetes
is treated by	insulin injections (plus a meal plan and careful monitoring)	diet first to reduce weight; oral medications to either stimulate more insulin production or make the available insulin work better; or insulin, if the first two methods are unsuccessful

changes in meal planning, and, in some cases, insulin injections. After the baby is born, the mother's pancreas usually begins functioning normally again. Although the infants of mothers with gestational diabetes are no more likely to develop type 1 diabetes than any other babies, women who have had gestational diabetes are at increased risk of developing type 2 diabetes later in life.

Finally, there are some less common types of diabetes that can occur in childhood. People with cystic fibrosis (CF) for example, can develop diabetes secondary to their CF, and some children who receive certain medications, such as glucocorticoids (e.g., cortisone, prednisone), may develop diabetes secondary to the medication. In such situations, the diabetes may go away once the medication is discontinued. Occasionally, diabetes may occur in families due to a single gene abnormality. When there is a strong family history of early onset type 2 diabetes, it may be important to search for these genetic conditions. In other words, when type 2 diabetes is diagnosed at a young age *and* there is a strong family history of the condition, then the chances of finding a single gene abnormality are more likely.

What Causes Type 1 Diabetes?

We do not know exactly why otherwise healthy people develop diabetes, but research has given us some clues. Type 1 diabetes is an autoimmune disorder, much like many thyroid disorders, rheumatoid arthritis, lupus, or multiple sclerosis. In these diseases, the body starts to see a part of itself as "foreign" and the immune system responds by destroying certain cells. In diabetes, the immune system destroys the insulin-producing beta cells. Researchers have so far identified two main factors behind this autoimmune response: genetics and environment.

Genetics

It appears that the susceptibility to develop type 1 diabetes is inherited, rather than the disease itself. This means that only some people born with a high level of susceptibility will actually develop the disorder. In fact, we find a history of other family members with type 1 diabetes in less than 10 percent of families. The fact that genetic factors can't be used to predict diabetes with 100 percent certainty suggests that other, presumably environmental factors may also be involved.

Risk of Developing Type 1 Diabetes If a Family Member Has It

Sibling (including non-identical twin)	1 in 20 chance
Identical twin	1 in 2–3 chance
Mother	1 in 50–100 chance
Father	1 in 16–20 chance
No family member	1 in 250–400 chance

Environment

The exact environmental trigger or triggers responsible for diabetes have not yet been determined. Some researchers believe that certain viral infections, illnesses, or environmental or food toxins may either damage the pancreas directly or trigger the autoimmune response. Other researchers have suggested that an increase in weight or BMI (body mass index) accelerates the development of type 1 diabetes. Many children diagnosed with diabetes have recently recovered from a virus or other illness. But everyone gets viruses and very few get diabetes. Although high levels of stress or even the onset of puberty frequently precedes the development of diabetes, stress is not generally believed to be the cause.

While diabetes is an autoimmune disorder, children with diabetes are no more susceptible to illness than any other child. Some people who have no personal experience of diabetes may be afraid that it's contagious, or may think of a child with diabetes as being "sick." Diabetes is not contagious. It cannot be passed on to another person through sharing a drink, playing together, kissing, or in any other way. Children with diabetes are just as healthy as their friends without it, once they have begun to manage the disease.

It's human nature to want to assign blame when something goes wrong. Many parents—and even children—are quick to blame the diabetes on themselves. Women sometimes fear they didn't take good enough care of themselves while pregnant; some worry their child ate too many sweets. But research shows that parents can't do anything to either cause or prevent diabetes. Nor can children. Children aren't born with type 1 diabetes, and at this stage we cannot yet predict with certainty who is going to get the disorder. And even if we could predict it, we would still have no way to prevent its onset.

What Does Insulin Do?

Insulin helps our bodies use glucose from the foods we eat, to make energy. We need energy to help make our muscles move, our heart beat, our lungs breath, our brain think—to do everything. That means we need insulin to survive.

How does insulin work with food? In a nutshell, here's what happens: When we eat, the food goes to the stomach and the small intestines where it is digested or broken down into components, or nutrients, small enough to be absorbed into the bloodstream and carried to every part of the body.

Food consists of three main nutrients: carbohydrate, protein, and fat. Our bodies derive energy from all three. Through digestion, carbohydrates (such as those in bread, potatoes, and fruit) are broken down into glucose; proteins (in foods such as meat and cheese) are converted into amino acids; and fats, including butter and oils, turn into fatty acids.

Glucose is an especially important source of energy, for two reasons—it can be converted quickly into energy when we need it, such as during work or sports; and the brain and nerves rely on a constant supply of glucose for their function.

In response to the glucose entering the bloodstream, the pancreas secretes insulin into the blood. Insulin stimulates the uptake of glucose by the cells of the body, so that they have the energy to do their work. Insulin also allows excess glucose to be stored in the liver, in the form of glycogen, or deposited in fat cells, where it becomes another important source of stored energy.

The insulin secreted by the pancreas in response to a meal is just the right amount to keep the blood glucose from going too high. After most of the nutrients from the meal have been taken up by the cells and the blood glucose concentration once again approaches "fasting" levels, the pancreas secretes less insulin into the blood.

Our body is almost always producing a small amount of insulin—called a basal amount. This is needed because, between meals and while we sleep, the liver continues to release some of its stored glucose into the blood, so that our brain and nerves receive the constant supply of glucose that they need to survive. This basal amount of insulin ensures that the balance between the amount of glucose being produced by the liver, and that being used by the cells of the body, is perfectly maintained to prevent either low or high glucose levels.

Later, when we eat again, another burst of insulin is secreted from the pancreas into the blood, and the liver stops releasing stored glucose and begins to replenish its stores for later use.

In summary: Insulin is an essential hormone. It acts as a key opening the door to the body's cells, allowing glucose to enter and to be used to make the energy so vital to their function. Without enough insulin, glucose cannot be taken up and used by most of the body's cells. The cells starve, even though the blood glucose concentration may be very high, and the body seeks alternate sources of energy. This leads eventually to the breakdown of fat and the production of harmful by-products called ketones.

Normal Blood Glucose Regulation

In Canada and many other places in the world, blood glucose is measured in units called millimoles of glucose per litre of blood (mmol/L). In the United States, blood glucose is measured in units called milligrams per decilitre or mg/dL; 1 mmol/L is equivalent to 18 mg/dL. So, for example, a blood glucose of 10 mmol/L is the same as a blood glucose of 180 mg/dL.

For someone without diabetes, the normal blood glucose level before breakfast (called fasting blood glucose), would be somewhere between 3.3 and 6 mmol/L (60–110 mg/dL). After eating, glucose levels will rise, but rarely above 8.9 mmol/L or 160 mg/dL, and never above 11.1 mmol/L or 200 mg/dL. Very small amounts of insulin are continuously released from the healthy pancreas. As soon as the blood glucose rises, a message to produce more insulin goes to the beta cells in the pancreas. The beta cells have sensors on their surface that detect the blood glucose level and give out just the right amount of insulin to handle the increased blood glucose.

When the blood glucose level comes down again, the burst of extra insulin shuts off. The beta cells keep a reserve of insulin on hand and, as that is used up, they produce more. So the

Turning food into energy: without diabetes

The stomach turns food into sugar.

The sugar is carried through the blood.

The pancreas makes enough
insulin to open the cell door.

Sugar enters the cell,
where it is used to make energy.

Turning food into energy: with diabetes

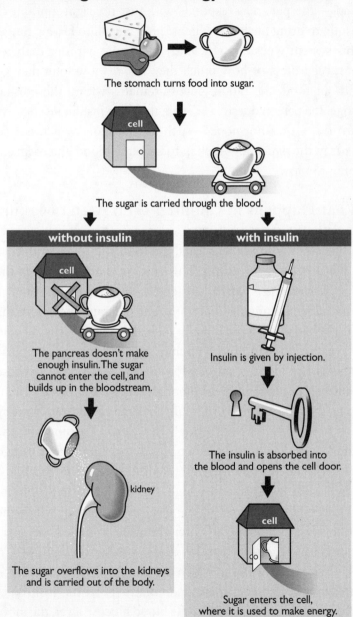

The stomach turns food into sugar.

The sugar is carried through the blood.

without insulin

The pancreas doesn't make enough insulin. The sugar cannot enter the cell, and builds up in the bloodstream.

kidney

The sugar overflows into the kidneys and is carried out of the body.

with insulin

Insulin is given by injection.

The insulin is absorbed into the blood and opens the cell door.

Sugar enters the cell, where it is used to make energy.

next time the person eats—be it a four-course meal or a quick snack—the pancreas responds with just the right amount of insulin to bring the blood glucose level back into fasting range. This system works so efficiently in people without diabetes that, regardless of how much they eat, or how long they go without food, the blood glucose remains within the normal range. If a person doesn't eat at all, the extra insulin just doesn't turn on. Other hormones—such as glucagon, which is also made in the pancreas—kick in to keep the blood glucose from going too low.

What Happens in Children Who Aren't Making or Taking Any Insulin?

As the child with diabetes eats, the food still releases glucose in the process of digestion. This glucose is absorbed into the bloodstream and is carried to the cells. But the pancreas doesn't respond by making insulin, so the glucose can't move into the cells. When the glucose remains locked out of the cells, a chain of events is set in motion. The child may become tired, because the cells are literally starved for energy. Meanwhile, glucose continues to build up in the blood. If this were allowed to continue, the blood would eventually become so thick and syrupy that it wouldn't flow through the veins. Fortunately, the kidneys do their job—to filter blood and eliminate, through the urine, substances that might otherwise harm the body.

When the kidneys sense a high level of glucose in the blood, they start eliminating it via the urine. The point at which the kidneys allow glucose to enter the urine is called the renal (kidney) threshold. When this excess glucose is eliminated, it takes with it the water in which it is dissolved, so the child urinates more often and in larger amounts (polyuria) just to get rid of the glucose. The higher the blood glucose level, the more frequent the urination. Increased urination leads to dehydration, so the body demands more water, and the child becomes increasingly thirsty (polydipsia). Children may complain of a dry sticky mouth or sore dry throat. Parents report children gulping down jugs of juice, and quantities of milk or water. Sometimes parents think the increased urination is caused by the excessive drinking so they try to cut off the fluids. However, the child continues to urinate frequently, because the body's priority is to clear out the excess glucose. Drinking all this fluid is the only way the child can avoid dehydration.

Excessive urination and thirst are usually the first indications of the high blood glucose (hyperglycemia) of diabetes. Often, children start getting up in the middle of the night to go to the bathroom (nocturia). Some may even start wetting the bed (enuresis). The loss of glucose in the urine, together with dehydration and the inability to use blood glucose, can lead to weight loss despite an increase in appetite (polyphagia). As the symptoms develop, children often feel tired, drowsy, and weak.

Using Fat for Energy
When Danny was admitted to hospital, his body was unable to make any, or enough, insulin to use glucose as energy. So where was he getting his energy? When the pancreas doesn't make insulin and the cells don't get their energy, the body starts to break down fat and proteins to be used as energy. When the body breaks down fat and protein, there is weight loss, which accounted for Danny's gaunt appearance. In the process of breaking down fat for energy, the body makes a potentially poisonous by-product called ketones, or acetone— the same chemical used in nail polish remover.

As soon as ketones are made, the kidneys recognize that they are poisonous and filter them out through the urine. Because Ruth didn't know her son had diabetes, she had no way of knowing that there were ketones present, or even what ketones were. Soon, Danny couldn't filter out the ketones as fast as they were being made, and they began to build up in his blood, leading to his stomachaches and severe nausea. This build-up of ketones is called diabetic ketoacidosis (DKA). When the body can't get rid of all the ketones through the urine, it can even resort to exhaling them, so that a fruity or unnatural smell may be noticeable on the child's breath. Danny's heavy, rapid breathing was his body's attempt to get rid of more ketones. This is called Kussmaul breathing.

Ketoacidosis is a serious condition that can lead to unconsciousness and death. Fortunately, giving intravenous fluid and insulin corrects the situation. In fact, this is the sickest most children with diabetes will ever be. Once a child has been diagnosed with diabetes, and the parents gain the tools and support they need to manage the disorder, diabetic ketoacidosis should be totally avoidable. Today diabetes is most often diagnosed before DKA has developed. The presence of the classic symptoms of diabetes should trigger further investigation in order to detect high glucose and ketones in the blood and/or urine before DKA has had time to develop.

While the earliest symptoms may be clear in older children, they may be less obvious in infants and toddlers. It's difficult to recognize thirst in young children who cannot speak. And regular growth spurts can bring changes in appetite. In these cases, therefore, the condition may quickly progress to DKA before it is recognized. An additional sign in those still in diapers may be a fungal or yeast diaper rash that doesn't improve with the use of medicated cream. These organisms flourish in the glucose excreted in the urine. In older girls, yeast infections (for example, vaginal discharge or itching) can also precede diagnosis.

Confirming the Diagnosis

Early Symptoms of Untreated or Undiagnosed Diabetes

Children with diabetes may:
- urinate a lot and often
- feel thirsty
- feel tired
- lose weight despite increased appetite

Danny's parents could hardly believe that, with one urine test and one blood test, their son was sentenced to living with diabetes. They thought that surely such a devastating diagnosis required a battery of tests to rule out other possibilities. The simple truth is that a urine test showing a lot of glucose as well as the presence of ketones, accompanied by symptoms such as excessive thirst and urination, establishes the diagnosis of diabetes. A reliable laboratory blood glucose reading of more than 11.1 mmol/L (200 mg/dL) taken at any time of day, regardless of when the child last ate, confirms it.

In children, making the distinction between type 1 and type 2 diabetes is usually not difficult. By far the majority of children and teens have type 1. Symptoms of type 1 diabetes usually have a dramatic onset because the pancreas stops making any insulin at all. Ketones are much more likely to be present in the urine in type 1 diabetes than in type 2. However, the absence of ketones doesn't mean that it isn't type 1; rather, it suggests that the child was diagnosed early, before ketones had the chance to form. Unfortunately, early diagnosis doesn't mean that the child has a less severe case of diabetes, or that treatment will be easier.

The child's symptoms disappear quite quickly once the insulin is replaced by injection. A few weeks after diagnosis, many parents are surprised to find that the insulin requirement decreases, giving the impression that the diabetes is going away. This is known as the remission, or the honeymoon period. During this time, the pancreas seems to be able to secrete some insulin, but this is only temporary. These changes in insulin dosage do not mean that the diabetes was misdiagnosed or that it has been cured. This period can last a few months or even a year or longer, but during that time the pancreas continues to lose insulin-producing cells. As the honeymoon comes to an end, the blood glucose rises and the daily insulin dose should increase, usually gradually, to an amount more consistent with what a child of that particular height and weight would require. This increase in insulin requirement should be seen as part of the natural course of the disease, rather than an indication that the diabetes is suddenly getting worse.

Type 2 Diabetes in Children and Adolescents

Although type 2 diabetes is much less common in children and adolescents, it seems to be increasing. Type 2 diabetes is much more likely to be found in adolescents than in younger children.

Certain risk factors predispose young people to the development of type 2 diabetes. These include:

- a strong family history of type 2 diabetes, especially if it developed in other family members at a young age
- obesity
- being a member of an ethnic group or population known to have a much higher prevalence of type 2 diabetes, such

as African American and African Canadian, Aboriginal American and Aboriginal Canadian, or Hispanic

As explained earlier, type 2 diabetes results from a combination of impaired insulin action in the muscle and fat cells of the body, and decreased insulin secretion from the pancreas. It is often associated with high blood fat (cholesterol and triglycerides) levels, high blood pressure, and a serious risk of later cardiovascular disease (heart attack or stroke).

Although the majority of adolescents with type 2 diabetes are considerably overweight, there are some who are thin, and the latter often have a strong family history of thin relatives developing type 2 diabetes at a young age. This type of diabetes is inherited as a dominant condition (that is, parents who have it may pass it on directly to half their children), and is called Maturity Onset Diabetes in the Young, or MODY.

In comparison to type 1 diabetes, type 2 diabetes usually begins with much milder symptoms, or without any symptoms at all. Occasionally, there is diabetic ketoacidosis (DKA), which can confuse the diagnosis.

The diagnosis of type 2 diabetes in adolescents is usually made after type 1 has been ruled out. Generally, when the young person has a strong history of symptoms, very high blood glucose readings, and ketones in the urine, type 1 diabetes is diagnosed. In adolescents with elevated blood glucose and only mild (or no) symptoms, no urinary ketones, and a strong family history of type 2 diabetes, type 2 diabetes is a possibility, but so is the early phase of type 1. Sometimes the doctor requests a blood test for islet cell antibodies. A positive result indicates type 1 diabetes; a negative result is inconclusive.

The initial management of type 2 diabetes depends on the blood glucose level and the severity of symptoms. Careful attention to meal planning is the cornerstone of treatment, and sometimes diet is enough to control the blood glucose. Of course, for an obese teen with type 2 diabetes an important goal of nutritional management is weight loss, which can be difficult. These young people need a supportive family environment as well as the help of a dietitian who understands adolescents. Most of them also need more physical activity. If, after several months, diet and exercise are not adequately controlling the blood glucose levels, medication may be required. Unlike type 1 diabetes, in which pills are of no benefit, in type 2, oral hypoglycemic agents (pills) such as sulfonylureas or biguanides are sometimes effective. These agents either stimulate the pancreas to produce more insulin, or help the cells of the body respond better to the insulin available. If blood glucose cannot be controlled with these agents, insulin treatment is necessary.

Young people with type 2 diabetes who have more severe symptoms and higher blood glucose readings usually need to take insulin injections in the beginning. As the blood glucose comes under control, the doctor will decide if oral hypoglycemic agents may be used in addition to, or instead of, the insulin.

This book focuses on the care of children and adolescents with type 1 diabetes. Although many of the concepts discussed apply to both types, young people diagnosed with type 2 diabetes should discuss possible differences, such as the role of exercise and the timing of meals, with their health care team.

Q&A

If the pancreas isn't working anymore, should it be removed?
No. Even if the beta cells are not producing insulin, the rest of the pancreas is still healthy and working. It is not a diseased organ, nor will it hinder the body in any other way. We know this because the pancreas also releases enzyme-rich juices that

aid in digestion, and children or teens with diabetes do not experience any unusual digestive problems. It also produces other hormones, such as glucagon, which may help protect against hypoglycemia.

Why can't insulin be administered by mouth?
Insulin is a protein hormone. Taken as a tablet or liquid, it would be broken down and digested in the stomach. However, insulin can't act unless it reaches the bloodstream before it's broken down. Therefore, it must be injected under the skin into an area of body fat. From there it is gradually absorbed into the bloodstream and transported to the cells.

When my uncle had a heart attack, the doctors discovered he had diabetes. He was on insulin for four or five years. Then, once he got his blood glucose under control, he didn't have to take it anymore. Is there a possibility my child might not need to take insulin after a while?
Unfortunately, there is no known cure for type 1 diabetes, and insulin administration, by injection or pump, remains the only way to manage it. Some people with type 2 diabetes, like your uncle, go on insulin to gain tighter control of their blood glucose during a particularly stressful period (such as after a heart attack) or until they've lost some weight. Eventually they may be able to keep good blood glucose control with diet alone or with pills.

My child has had diabetes for three weeks now, and it seems that our whole lives revolve around the disease. Is this going to go on forever?
The way you're feeling right now is normal and necessary. Learning about diabetes, and adjusting to it, should be your priority. The immediate impact of the disorder is overwhelming

for all members of the family. Try to take one day at a time, and don't be afraid to lean on your diabetes team for support and guidance. As time goes on, you will feel more comfortable with the daily routines of diabetes care. But be patient; it can take a year or perhaps longer before you go a day without worrying about your child's condition.

How will I know if one of my other children is developing diabetes?

The table earlier in the chapter shows the likelihood of others in the family developing diabetes. If this should happen in one of your other children, he or she will almost certainly start to show such "classic" symptoms as increased urination and thirst, and weight loss. If you are concerned, simply do a urine test for glucose. If there is no glucose present, it's not diabetes. If there is glucose present, contact your family doctor or diabetes team immediately.

What should my child say when people ask why she was away from school?

It's often difficult for children to know what and when to tell classmates. Other children may be scared, too. Tell them that diabetes is not contagious. To anyone who wants to know more, or anyone with whom your child wishes to share her condition, you can say that diabetes simply means that your child's body needs help making energy from food. Your child needs to take insulin injections because her body stopped making its own insulin. Involve your child's friends in her diabetes routines, if they want to learn and if you and your child are comfortable showing them. Your child may even want to prepare a presentation or science project about diabetes.

TWO

Striking a Balance

Phil and Arlene are very proud of their daughter Jenny. At age 14, just one year after being diagnosed with diabetes, Jenny has taken on many of the responsibilities of monitoring and treating her own condition. She checks her blood glucose four times a day, prepares and injects her needles, and follows her daily meal plan by careful carbohydrate counting and eating at about the same times every day. Every night Arlene checks Jenny's diabetes log to make sure she's keeping track. Jenny carefully records how much insulin she takes and when, and color-codes the results of her glucose tests according to the level: red for over 8 mmol/L (145 mg/dL); green for her target range of 4 to 8 mmol/L (70–145 mg/dL); and blue for under 4 mmol/L (70 mg/dL). The logbook pages of the past month are mostly green, except for a few numbers in red and three or four in blue.

Jenny has had no low blood glucose readings that she hasn't been able to handle. A couple of times she got shaky after a vigorous game of soccer. Fortunately, she remembered to boost her blood glucose with a little juice (she always carries a juice box in her knapsack) and she felt fine after just a couple of minutes.

Jenny loves school too much to miss it, and her teacher recently commented that she hadn't thought about Jenny's diabetes in months. Arlene wishes she could say the same. Even though she worries less about Jenny now than during those first few months, it's always in the back of her mind. Jenny has diabetes. Arlene has to remind herself that, unless medical science finds a way to overcome the disease, Jenny will always have diabetes.

Balanced blood sugar

The Concept of Blood Glucose Balance

Blood glucose levels go up and down throughout the day. Think of a teeter-totter. When you eat, blood glucose goes up. When you exercise, blood glucose goes down. In people without diabetes, insulin automatically accommodates these fluctuations. People with diabetes inject insulin in an attempt to mimic the body's natural insulin production as closely as possible. However, injected insulin cannot perfectly match the fluctuations in blood glucose, so someone with diabetes has to work constantly to keep the teeter-totter from tipping.

The goal of diabetes management is to restore and maintain blood glucose balance. The first step is to eliminate any symptoms of high blood glucose with insulin injections. The next step is to match the child's appetite and dietary needs for growth and development with the amount of insulin injected. As children grow and develop and as their lifestyle and activities change, so do their insulin needs.

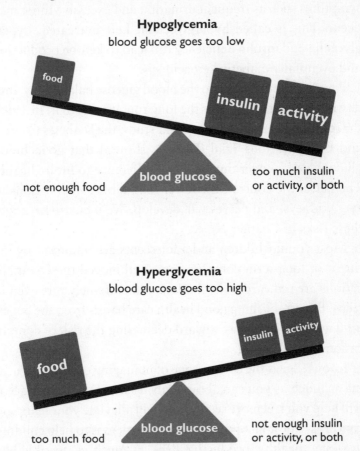

Hypoglycemia
blood glucose goes too low

not enough food   blood glucose   too much insulin or activity, or both

Hyperglycemia
blood glucose goes too high

too much food   blood glucose   not enough insulin or activity, or both

Blood glucose balance is important to immediate and long-term health. There are two immediate consequences of blood glucose imbalance. If the blood glucose level dips too low (usually below 3–4 mmol/L or 55–70 mg/dL), the child can become shaky, hungry, tired, or grouchy. Eventually, if no glucose is given, the child may become confused or unconscious. This is called hypoglycemia. If the blood glucose level climbs too high (usually above 11 mmol/L, or 200 mg/dL), symptoms such as frequent urination and excessive thirst may occur. This is called hyperglycemia. Left untreated, hyperglycemia and insulin deficiency can lead to ketone production and eventually diabetic ketoacidosis.

Paying close attention to the blood glucose balance day after day is hard work. But over the long run, it's worth it. In 1993, the results of a landmark nine-year study, the Diabetes Control and Complications Trial (DCCT), showed that good blood glucose control over time makes a difference to future health. The better the control, the fewer long-term complications to eyes, kidneys, and nerves will develop. We'll talk more about these risks in Chapter Nine.

Most young children and adolescents are unmoved by the threat of long-term complications, and indeed these complications are unheard of in children and extremely rare even in teens. But establishing good health care habits from the beginning will go a long way toward decreasing the risk of complications in adulthood.

Knowledge is the cornerstone of managing diabetes. Learning as much as you can about diabetes and how to manage it will help you feel more secure, and will alleviate your fears and concerns. The goal of diabetes management is to help children live long, healthy, productive lives, as much as possible like any other child.

Gaining Control

Before looking down the road into adulthood, children with diabetes and their parents need to figure out how to live with diabetes from day to day. Children with good diabetes control can be expected to enjoy good general physical and emotional well-being, characterized by:

- no symptoms of high blood glucose levels (i.e., increased urination and thirst)
- only mild and infrequent low blood glucose reactions
- normal growth and physical development
- lots of energy
- interest in friends and activities
- regular school attendance

Factors That Affect Blood Glucose Balance

Insulin and food have a major impact on blood glucose level. The carbohydrates in the food we eat increase our blood glucose. Insulin lowers the blood glucose level by allowing glucose to enter the cells, where it's used for energy. In order to achieve healthy blood glucose levels people with type 1 diabetes need to strike a balance between the food they eat and the insulin they inject.

Insulin

In people without diabetes, the pancreas delivers tiny amounts of insulin continuously and secretes extra insulin when food enters the system in order to counteract the increase in blood glucose. Injected insulin performs a similar function. Traditionally, young children have started out with two or three injections of insulin each day (before breakfast, supper, and bed). This routine may work for some. For others, especially after the honeymoon, multiple daily insulin injections (MDI) or a continuous infusion of insulin delivered under the skin by an insulin pump are generally being recommended. Insulin pump therapy can be used for children of all ages. These newer methods of replacing insulin make sense in many ways, since they more closely mimic the way our bodies release insulin, therefore better blood glucose control may be achieved.

Food

It's important for children with diabetes to maintain a healthy level of blood glucose, by matching their food intake with the appropriate amount of insulin. There are different ways to accomplish this. Children taking two or three injections are generally required to be on a routine where they eat similar amounts of food at about the same time each day. Only then is insulin action predictable. Children on multiple daily injections with rapid-acting insulin with meals and snacks or a continuous insulin infusion system (insulin pump), frequently learn how much insulin they need to take in order to balance the carbohydrate content of individual meals and snacks. The routine of carbohydrate counting and frequent injections is more work in some ways but this system has the potential for increased flexibility without compromising the blood glucose balance.

When there is a mismatch between food and insulin the child runs the risk of high or low blood glucose levels. If there isn't enough glucose in the body to work with the insulin, the child may experience low blood sugar or hypoglycemia and signs of an "insulin reaction." Conversely, if there is too much food for the given amount of insulin, high blood sugar or hyperglycemia will result.

Most parents agree that meal planning and getting the food/insulin balance is the biggest challenge in managing diabetes. A dietitian will help you to create a meal plan for your child, keeping in mind family habits and favorite foods. The goal is not to restrict food or calories, but to ensure healthy eating and to remain consistent enough to be able to determine the insulin dosage.

Other Factors Affecting Glucose Control

In our discussions about diabetes management we focus a great deal on insulin replacement and meal planning because these components of the treatment program have a big impact on blood glucose levels and because the child and parents have control over how much insulin is taken and how much food is eaten. But no matter how hard you try to match food with the insulin, the results of the blood glucose readings will vary. Why? Injected insulin can't match the automatic response of a normal pancreas. And there are other factors that affect blood glucose, which may be more difficult to control, particularly in children, such as activity and stress.

Activity

Activity in the presence of insulin lowers the blood glucose level, because when the body burns more energy it uses more glucose. An active lifestyle is an important aspect of good health. It improves physical fitness, helps us relax, and promotes general well-being. A child's diabetes care routine should take into account the amount of exercise or activity he or she experiences on a daily basis. Parents, and eventually the child, will learn to adjust the routines for special activities.

For people with diabetes, exercise offers an additional advantage. It helps improve the action of a given amount of insulin, so that less insulin may be needed to maintain the blood glucose level. For example, an active person requires less insulin than someone watching television, because activity brings blood glucose down. Regular exercise also seems to make muscles and other tissues more responsive to insulin, so the body requires less insulin to move glucose from the blood into the muscles. As well, regular exercise may help decrease the risk of diabetes complications.

These benefits aside, exercise and activity must not be considered a tool of diabetes treatment. Children generally lead naturally active lives; turning exercise into something "prescribed" takes the fun away. A positive example from parents is essential. Exercise and activity should be part of an enjoyable family routine. That's not to say that everyone with diabetes has to become a competitive athlete, but children should participate in sports and physical activity at their own level.

How Exercise Affects Blood Glucose

In general, activity causes the muscles to draw more glucose from the blood. In people without diabetes, the pancreas makes and secretes much less insulin, the liver produces more glucose for the body to use, and the level of glucose in the blood remains steady.

In children with diabetes, the injected insulin is unable to "shut off." The muscles continue to use up the available glucose in the blood. If the insulin is injected into an arm or leg in someone who has been particularly active, such as playing tag or bicycling, there may in fact be an increase in the flow of insulin absorbed from the injection site into the blood. This insulin causes the muscles to draw more glucose, prevents the liver from replenishing the supply of glucose in the blood, and may therefore put the child at risk of a low blood glucose reaction.

While most activities lead to a decrease in blood glucose levels, some very stressful or competitive activities (such as ice hockey or soccer) may increase the glucose levels, because the heavy stress of the game increases "stress" hormones that work against the insulin. Sometimes, too, the glucose level doesn't fall during the activity, especially if it occurs immediately after a meal. However, the glucose may then drop for up to 6 to 12 hours after the activity is over. This means that children doing strenuous activity in the late afternoon or evening may be susceptible to late-night "lows."

Stress

Stress generally increases the blood glucose level. Stress is the body's physical response to danger, left over from the days when we had to fight natural predators for survival. Though the causes of stress may have changed through the ages, the body's reaction has not. Stress triggers a surge of power-boosting hormones, such as adrenaline and glucagon. These hormones in turn stimulate the release into the blood of glucose stored in the liver and muscles as glycogen. Because children with diabetes do not automatically make more insulin to deal with this, they end up with a high blood glucose level.

Today's stress can be emotional, caused by exams or peer pressure, for example, or physical, accompanying fever and infection. Stress can also come in the form of excitement over seeing friends and family, or anticipating a special occasion. The bottom line is that sometimes stress makes the blood glucose go up temporarily. During a stressful event like an illness, parents and child will need to check blood glucose levels more frequently and take appropriate action.

Parents do not need to make any special attempt to create a "stress-free" environment for their child. Checking blood glucose regularly and making adjustments based on the results will help maintain the blood glucose balance.

Checking Blood Glucose Balance

Checking the blood glucose level several times each day is the best way to determine how well the child with diabetes is balancing insulin, food, and activity.

The diabetes health care team works with the family to determine a blood glucose range that fits each child's age and stage of development. No matter how hard the parents and child try to monitor meals and snacks, how carefully they stick to insulin regimens or how active they may be, not every reading will fall into this range. In fact, in the beginning, very few may be in target. It is not unusual for parents or children to feel they have done something "wrong" or "bad" if levels are off target. But try to avoid looking at each blood glucose check as a report card; rather, see it as a piece of a road map that helps you make appropriate decisions about diabetes management.

Q&A

I read somewhere that, after they're diagnosed with type 1 diabetes, people can become overweight. Is this true?
Not really. When diabetes develops there is usually some weight loss (sometimes just a little, other times quite a lot). With treatment the lost weight will soon be regained. Otherwise, young people with type 1 diabetes, particularly teenage girls, are only slightly more likely than their non-diabetic peers to become overweight. Getting or remaining active and using an insulin regimen that allows for a careful match between food and insulin will also promote a healthy weight.

My daughter isn't very active. I'd like to get her involved in something physical, to avoid increasing her insulin. What can you suggest?

It's great that you want to encourage your daughter to get more involved in physical fitness, but remember, exercise is not therapy. If she preferred books to baseball before she had diabetes, there's no reason to expect her to suddenly change. Nevertheless, encourage her to participate in physical activities. Activity should be fun. You might start with family walks and go on to other social activities she likes, such as dancing, bicycling, swimming, or tennis.

Why doesn't exercise always help bring down high blood glucose?
In general, exercise does help lower the blood glucose level. But once blood glucose is very high—for example, over 17 mmol/L (300 mg/dL)—don't count on exercise to bring it down. The only thing sure to bring it down is insulin. Strenuous exercise without enough insulin prompts the liver to release stored glucose, which in turn increases blood glucose. In someone with high blood glucose and not enough insulin, the glucose just keeps building up. Don't exercise if you are ill and urine ketones are present.

Why does my son's blood glucose always go sky-high after exercise?
There are two reasons this may happen. First, if his diabetes is poorly controlled, so that he has frequent high blood glucose readings, exercise will be a further stress causing even higher glucose. Secondly, in some children with well-controlled diabetes, very strenuous exercise can cause stress and increased glucose levels. They may not need extra food to cover the exercise, but may need more insulin. In such situations, beware of late-night lows.

My daughter was very sick with diabetic ketoacidosis at the time she was diagnosed. How can I be sure that she will never get sick like that again?

Once children are diagnosed with diabetes and established on insulin, there are really only two reasons why they might develop diabetic ketoacidosis again, and both are preventable. First, an illness such as a fever, infection, or flu may create a demand for more insulin than normal. If you don't realize this and make the appropriate adjustments, DKA may result. (See "Sick Days," in Chapter Six.)

Secondly, failure to take any or enough insulin will result in DKA. As long as you are in charge of giving the insulin, this is unlikely. However, when children are left to inject their own insulin unsupervised before they have developed sound judgment (or when an illness impairs their judgment), DKA may result when they forget, or even intentionally neglect, to inject the insulin. Wise parents remain involved in supporting and supervising their children with injections long into their adolescent years. As children become more independent, parents should watch for warning signs that things are not going well— for example, a recurrence of the symptoms of hyperglycemia, such as weight loss or polyuria or of ketones in the urine. When parents notice these signs they should resume close supervision, or even give the insulin injections for a while, regardless of their child's age.

THREE

All about Insulin

It has been six months since Margie was diagnosed with diabetes. She's a fun-loving, active four-year-old who has adjusted well, except to the insulin injections. She's great with the finger prick for blood glucose. She even applies the drop of blood to the strip. But when it comes to the injection, she kicks up a fuss. The shot before breakfast is especially hard for Margie and her parents, John and Liz. It's a hectic time: her brothers and sisters are busy getting ready for school, Mom and Dad are trying to get off to work, and Margie throws a temper tantrum. John is just as happy to back off, since he hates giving Margie her injections anyway, which means Liz has to step in and get the needle over with. These episodes are wearing the family's patience thin, and not helping Margie either. "Try making it less of an ordeal," suggests their diabetes nurse when Liz calls in desperation one morning. "Draw the insulin, prepare the syringe, and get everything ready before Margie even comes downstairs for breakfast." The nurse recommends that both John and Liz be present for the injection, to show Margie they are there for her, and to take some of the stress off Liz. It helps for one parent to hold Margie while the other gives the injection. Letting Margie hold a special stuffed toy may also comfort her.

Despite the long history of diabetes, no real headway was made in the understanding or treatment of the disease until 1889. German physiologists Oskar Minkowski and Joseph von Mering learned, quite accidentally, that the pancreas was central to diabetes. In studying digestion in a laboratory dog, they removed the pancreas to see the effect. When the dog started urinating more often than usual, the doctors tested the urine for glucose. Indeed, the dog had the markers of diabetes. In 1893, scientist Paul Langerhans isolated cells in the pancreas (the islets of Langerhans) that produced a hormone, but doctors still didn't understand its function.

As doctors inched closer to finding a treatment, young people with diabetes still didn't fare well. Most died within a year of diagnosis. In 1921, the breakthrough came when a young surgeon at the University of Toronto, Dr. Frederick Banting, and his student, Charles Best, focused on the unknown hormone produced in the islets of Langerhans.

Still working with dogs, Banting and Best limited pancreatic function by tying off the ducts that send digestive enzymes from the pancreas into the intestine. The theory was that the islet cells, which secrete the hormone into the bloodstream, wouldn't be affected. Banting isolated a substance from these cells and injected it into a diabetic dog. The success was not immediate, but eventually Banting and Best treated the dog with the islet extract, soon to be labeled "insulin" (from the Latin word "insula," meaning "island").

The real test, of course, was a human subject. Leonard Thompson, a 14-year-old boy dying of diabetes, was confined to his bed. He was little more than paper-thin skin wrapped around a skeleton. The first injection of insulin had no effect. A biochemist purified the canine insulin, and after twelve days of treatment the boy began to look like himself again. (Thompson eventually died of pneumonia at age 29.) Two years after their landmark discovery, Banting and Professor J.J.R. MacLeod (in whose lab the experiments took place) were awarded the Nobel Prize in Physiology and Medicine. Banting subsequently shared his prize with Best, while MacLeod recognized the efforts of the biochemist J.B. Collip.

Types of Insulin

Initially manufacturers used cows and pigs to produce insulin. These insulin preparations are no longer available and since 1983 biosynthetic human insulin has been available. This is produced in a laboratory by introducing a synthetic human gene into bacteria or yeast, which produces insulin identical in structure and function to that created in the human pancreas. Through further modifications, manufacturers can prepare insulins (called insulin analogs) with different action times.

Action

Manufactured insulin is generally categorized into four groups: rapid-acting lispro (Humalog), aspart (NovoRapid) and glulisine (Apidra), short-acting (regular or soluble), intermediate-acting isophane (NPH), and long-acting glargine (Lantus) and detemir (Levemir). Insulin preparations are also described according to their course of action: *onset* is the time taken for the insulin to start working, *peak* describes the period when the insulin is working at its strongest, and *duration* describes the length of time before the effect of the dose wears off. Taken right before a meal, rapid-acting insulin begins to work within 5 to 10 minutes and helps to control the rise in blood glucose immediately after eating. Intermediate and longer-acting insulin analogs such as Lantus and Levemir reduce the blood glucose levels throughout the day and night.

Insulin's Effect: How Soon, How Long

	Appearance	Onset	Peak	Duration
Rapid (Humalog, NovoRapid, Apidra*)	clear	5–10 min.	first 2 hours	3–4 hours
Short (Regular, Toronto)	clear	1/2–1 hour	2–4 hours	4–6 hours
Intermediate (NPH)	cloudy	2–4 hours	6–12 hours	18–24 hours
Long (Lantus, Levemir)	cloudy	4 hours	minimal peak	20–30 hours

These times represent averages for each preparation, and may vary from person to person, from one injection site to another, and to some extent in the same person from day to day.

*Apidra is not yet licensed in Canada for children. Approval for children aged 4 and over is expected in 2010/11. Check with your doctor.

Insulin Strength

In North America, insulin is dispensed in a concentration of 100 units/1 mL. It's available in bottles to be used with syringes and in cartridges that are used with insulin pens and with some brands of insulin pumps. Each bottle of insulin holds 10 mL, or 1,000 units. Pen cartridges hold 3 mL or 300 units.

Buying Insulin

Insulin is sold in any pharmacy and in most places it's available without a prescription. Each bottle or cartridge has an expiry date (usually one to two years after the purchase date). The insulin bottle should be discarded after that date.

Each 10 mL bottle of insulin costs roughly US$20–$75, or C$25–$75 depending on the type of insulin. Pen cartridges cost more per unit of insulin. Insulin purchase is covered by some provincial government health care plans in Canada, and most insurance companies require a prescription in order to reimburse the cost.

Manufacturers of Insulin
Eli Lilly, Novo Nordisk, and sanofi-aventis are the major manufacturers of insulin in North America. A list of available products is provided in the Table of Insulin Types at the end of this book.

Care of Insulin
Insulin can be kept safely in the refrigerator until its expiry date. After opening, most insulin preparations can be stored at room temperature for a month—slightly less for glargine (28 days).

Insulin is a very stable substance that doesn't go bad easily. However, if it is allowed to freeze or get extremely hot, it can be damaged. If a clear insulin preparation becomes cloudy or straw-colored, or if it has solid particles floating in it, it should not be used. With cloudy insulin preparations, such as NPH, it is natural for the white substance to settle to the bottom of the bottle over a period of time. This should mix easily into the solution. Don't use cloudy insulin if particles or lumps are floating around after mixing, or if solid pieces stick to the bottom or side of the bottle. To be safe, if the insulin is exposed to an extreme temperature, discard the bottle.

When hiking, camping, or traveling long distances, it is important to protect bottles from breakage and temperature extremes. You can do this by wrapping them individually and placing them in a small thermal container. Those involved in winter sports, such as skiing or winter camping, are wise to prevent the insulin (and the tubing for the insulin pump) from freezing by keeping it close to the body. Always keep a spare bottle of insulin on hand in case one gets damaged. For children using two kinds of insulin, keep a spare bottle of each type.

Injecting Insulin

Often, for the parents of children who have been newly diagnosed, injecting their child with insulin is the biggest hurdle to overcome. Many are squeamish about needles, never mind giving one to their own child. Teenagers, and indeed some younger children, quickly become quite adept at administering their own insulin. Initially, however, both parents need to become proficient, too. Other caregivers such as grandparents and babysitters should also be able to give an injection in case of illness or emergency. Children who are preparing and injecting their own insulin must be supervised to ensure that the dose is accurate, the insulin is actually injected, and the child doesn't favor the same injection site day after day. Supervision will remind them that insulin is important, and potentially dangerous if too much is given at one time. When both parents are involved, the mutual support encourages better family adaptation to diabetes.

Injecting with a Syringe and Needle

At first, parents and children learn to inject insulin with a syringe specifically designed to measure insulin. The syringe has three parts: the needle, the plunger, and the barrel.

Insulin syringes are generally available in four sizes: 1/4 mL or 25 units, 3/10 mL or 30 units, 1/2 mL or 50 units, and 1 mL or 100 units. All are intended to measure 100 units per mL insulin, which is the standard strength available in North America. The larger the dose, the larger the syringe.

Syringes

Needles are available in a variety of lengths and thicknesses, and are measured in gauges. The higher the gauge number, the finer the needle. The needle on insulin syringes comes in two standard lengths: 1/2 inch (12.8 mm) or 3/8 inch (8 mm). Pen needles are as short as 1/4 inch (5 or 6 mm). Generally, children prefer finer needles because they hurt less. While shorter needles may be more comfortable for younger or thinner children, teenagers may choose slightly longer needles to avoid a painful lump under the skin and to ensure the insulin is injected at the right depth.

Preparing a Single Type of Insulin

Using an Insulin Syringe
- Wash your hands. Gather together the insulin and the syringe.
- Double-check the label on the insulin to make sure you have the right kind.
- Note the expiry date.

- For cloudy insulin preparations, roll the bottle gently between your hands for 5 to 10 seconds to mix it thoroughly. Do not shake the bottle, or the insulin will become frothy and difficult to measure.
- Make sure the insulin is uniformly mixed, or the dose administered may vary greatly.
- Remove the cover from the needle.
- Pull back on the plunger to draw up air. You will need as many units of air as the units of insulin you will be injecting. If you are planning to inject 20 units of insulin, draw 20 units of air into the syringe.
- With the insulin bottle right side up, insert the needle into the rubber stopper on top of the bottle and push the plunger down so the air enters the top of the bottle. This equalizes the pressure and prevents a vacuum in the bottle, making it easier to withdraw the insulin. Avoid injecting air into the insulin itself.
- Leaving the needle in the bottle, turn the bottle upside down, making sure the tip of the needle is fully immersed in the insulin. Do not draw air into the syringe.
- Pull back the plunger to the number of units of insulin required. Ensure there are no air bubbles in the syringe, because they would take up space where insulin should be.
- Remove any air bubbles by flicking the syringe with your finger until they rise to the top. You may need to push the plunger upward to get rid of the air and then reset the plunger at the correct number of units. If the air is not removed, the dose will not be adequate.
- Whenever possible, double-check with another person that you have the correct kind and amount of insulin in the syringe.
- Take the needle out of the bottle and replace the cap if you are going to be moving to another room to do the injection. With younger children, these steps can be taken in a different room to create less disruption for the child.

Giving the Injection

- Gather together the insulin-loaded syringe and a dry cotton swab or tissue.
- Select the injection site. (See p. 46.)
- Gently pinch up the skin and fat with the thumb and fore-finger.
- Hold the syringe like a pencil, close to the needle for better control.
- Push the needle in quickly and all the way, at a 90-degree angle to the pinched-up skin.
- Push the plunger in to inject the insulin.
- Slowly let go of the pinched-up skin and then remove the needle.
- Using a dry swab, apply gentle pressure to the injection site to prevent bruising.
- Discard the needle and syringe in a special container, available at your pharmacy, or recycle a juice can or empty bleach container. To avoid possible injury, never leave used needles lying around.

Preparing a Mixture of Insulin Types

Using an Insulin Syringe

Some young people take two different types of insulin mixed in one injection. This is possible when the youngster is on a combination of short-acting or rapid-acting insulin (regular, lispro, or aspart) to work with the food in the coming meal, and intermediate-acting insulin (NPH) that will peak later in the day.

Preparing an injection of two types of insulin is similar to preparing an injection of one type. The only difference is that you prepare both bottles of insulin (rolling the cloudy insulin, and injecting the appropriate amounts of air into each bottle) and then draw up the prescribed amounts from each bottle.

- Put as many units of air into the bottle of intermediate (cloudy) insulin as you plan to draw out in insulin, but do not withdraw the insulin yet.
- Remove the needle from the bottle of cloudy insulin, and put as many units of air into the bottle of the clear or rapid-acting insulin as you plan to draw out in insulin. Go ahead and withdraw the prescribed amount of clear insulin.
- Make sure there are no large air bubbles.
- Now add the prescribed amount of the cloudy, intermediate-acting insulin to the same syringe.
- If you accidentally pull the plunger back too far when adding the second kind of insulin, discard the insulin in the syringe and begin again. If clear insulin is mixed into the cloudy insulin bottle by mistake, discard that bottle.
- Once the correct dose of insulin is prepared, inject as usual.

You can also withdraw the intermediate-acting insulin first, followed by the short-acting or rapid-acting insulin.

Injecting with Pens and Cartridges

A method of injection that is often more convenient than a syringe is the insulin pen. Rather than withdrawing insulin from a bottle, you use a cartridge of insulin that fits into a pen-like device that has a special needle tip that screws onto the end of the pen. By turning the dial on the side of the pen, you can set the dose. When you push down on the end of the pen (like a plunger) the insulin is delivered. Each 3 mL cartridge holds 300 units of insulin. With some insulin pens you are able to measure doses in half-unit increments, a feature that is important for young children requiring tiny doses. Pen needle tips are available in three sizes: regular length (12.8 mm), short (8 mm), and a mini length (5 or 6 mm). Regardless of the needle size, many children find that pen injections hurt less than syringes, probably because the needle never has to go through the rubber stopper of an insulin bottle, and so stays sharper. Pen injections are also more portable and discreet, and quicker to prepare, than insulin injections by syringe. The main drawback is that many children are on a combination of insulins, at least in the morning, and pens are designed to give only a single type of insulin at a time. All the same, pen injections are the insulin delivery devices of choice for most children at times of the day when they are receiving only one kind of insulin. Some may even choose to use two separate pens, rather than combining two kinds of insulin in a syringe.

There are some important technical differences between using a pen and using a syringe. Here are some tips for using the pen accurately. If your child is experiencing erratic blood glucose control, it is a good idea to assess each of these steps carefully.

- Insulin cartridges should have no air in them. To mix the cloudy insulin, gently invert the cartridge at least twenty times. The up-and-down movement of a glass bead in the cartridge will help the insulin achieve uniform suspension.
- Before you give each injection, satisfy yourself that the device is working: check for insulin flow by squirting 2 units in the air. Keep doing this until you see insulin come out of the needle.
- If you use a mini needle (5 mm), do not pinch up the skin. Doing so may result in insulin leaking back.
- After injecting the insulin, count to five slowly before removing the needle. If you miss this step, you may not be giving the whole dose.
- Remove the needle from the pen or cartridge immediately after injecting. If you leave the needle on, you may introduce air into the cartridge and/or insulin may leak out. Both may lead to an inaccurate insulin dose.

Selecting the Injection Site When Using Syringes and Pens
There are four safe areas for insulin injections.

- Thighs: top and outer areas only. Do not use the inner side or back of the thigh, and stay about four of the child's finger-widths away from the knee and groin.
- Upper arms: fleshy area on the side and back of the arms. Avoid the muscle in the shoulder, and stay three to four finger-widths away from the elbow.
- Abdomen: right across the abdomen, from just below the ribcage to well below the belt line. Stay about two finger-widths away from the navel.
- Buttocks: fleshy area (e.g., jeans' pocket area).

Injection sites

Insulin may be absorbed differently from one site than from another. Absorption is most predictable when injections are given in the abdomen and buttocks. In general, insulin injected into the upper arms or thighs is absorbed more erratically. Also, insulin injected over an exercising muscle may be absorbed more quickly, so it's wise to avoid injecting into the arms or thighs of someone who's planning strenuous exercise including these muscles (i.e., runners should avoid injections into the thighs, rowers should avoid injections into the arms, and so on).

Injections are done in a pattern, to avoid using exactly the same site over and over. Ensure that each injection is about 1 inch (2.5 cm) or two finger-widths from the previous one. Try to work in straight, even rows about an inch apart. Stay in one site for seven to fourteen days, ensuring appropriate spacing between injections. This way you're more likely to remember where the last injection was given.

Rotating Injection Sites

Many people with diabetes, children especially, develop "favorite" injection sites where the pain seems to be less and injections seem easier. If the same small area is used repeatedly, the fat tissue below the skin swells (lipohypertrophy), creating large bumps that absorb insulin poorly. They may go away in time when the site is left alone. Until the bumps have disappeared, inject into another area to promote better insulin absorption. Sometimes repeated injections into the same site do not produce lipohypertrophy, but rather a hard area of scar tissue under the skin. These sites should also be avoided. At each clinic visit a member of the diabetes team will examine the injection areas to help with site selection and the prevention of lumps or bumps.

Insulin Pumps

Continuous subcutaneous (beneath the skin) insulin infusion pumps (insulin pumps) are another way of giving insulin. These devices have become more and more popular. When used correctly, an insulin pump more closely mimics a normally functioning pancreas and allows a child to lead a more normal and flexible lifestyle. The pump offers the potential for excellent blood glucose control with less hypoglycemia, particularly overnight. It also allows for more flexibility in a child's food choices, exercise, and sleeping. When used very thoughtfully, children using the pump are sometimes able to achieve better blood glucose control than children using other systems of insulin delivery.

How Do Insulin Pumps Work?

The pump delivers a steady trickle of rapid-acting insulin 24 hours a day. This basal insulin keeps the blood glucose level under control during times of the day and night when there is no food intake, and protects the body from ketone production. However, basal insulin does not provide coverage for meals or snacks. The user has to program the pump to give insulin with food by pushing a button on the pump to deliver a "bolus," or surge of rapid-acting insulin just before food intake. The bolus dose can be adjusted for the person's glucose level, the carbohydrate content of the meal, and the activity they are planning after the meal.

A pump is about the size of a pager, and can be worn on a belt or carried in a pocket. The pump delivers insulin through a small plastic tube or cannula that is inserted under the skin, usually on the abdomen, or the buttocks, and then taped in place. A length of fine, flexible tubing connects the cannula to the pump. The cannula stays in place for about three days. It is then removed and a new cannula is inserted at a new site.

Who Can Use an Insulin Pump?

Anybody with diabetes can potentially benefit from an insulin pump. Children are now starting to use the pump at younger ages, and sooner after diagnosis. In fact, even babies with diabetes can be treated with an insulin pump.

Perfect control of diabetes is not a requirement for using the pump. Many children make significant improvements in blood glucose control once they are using an insulin pump.

Success depends on both good family support and commitment on the part of the youngster with diabetes to make insulin pump therapy work. Good candidates for the insulin pump also:

- come to clinic regularly
- are comfortable with diabetes and willing to let others know that they have diabetes
- are knowledgeable about diabetes
- are confident in carbohydrate counting
- are prepared to do six to ten blood glucose tests per day, at least during the first few weeks
- have good attention to detail and good decision-making and problem-solving skills

If you think that you and your child can learn to use the pump successfully, speak to your diabetes team.

What Are the Advantages of Insulin Pumps?

- For some individuals it is easier to achieve good blood glucose control with a pump. You can adjust and manage insulin levels more precisely, with careful and frequent monitoring. Insulin pumps allow you to more closely mimic the normal action of a healthy pancreas.
- Pumps can help people achieve better long-term control as evidenced by a lower A1C—a measure of average blood glucose concentrations taken during the previous three months. Pumps may also reduce fluctuation between high

and low blood glucose concentrations and pump use is generally associated with a lower risk of hypoglycemia.
- The child only needs one needle poke about every three days to insert the new cannula. A push of a button delivers extra insulin when needed.
- The pump can be very liberating. Initially, learning to use the pump takes some time. However, subsequently the child has much more freedom and flexibility to eat, sleep, and exercise when she wants.
- Improved blood glucose control reduces the risk of complications down the road.

What Are the Disadvantages of Insulin Pumps?
- Because the pump delivers only rapid-acting insulin, there are no long-acting insulin reserves to fall back on if there is a problem. This means that blood glucose and ketone levels can rise very quickly if something goes wrong with the pump or the insertion site. Blood glucose levels must be monitored more often.
- Insulin pumps and pump supplies are expensive. Not all private health insurance plans pay for these. In 2006, in Ontario, Canada, the provincial government began paying for pumps and pump supplies for children and teens with type 1 diabetes, who meet specific criteria. Subsequently, the program was expanded to include adults with type 1 diabetes.
- Some people find the pump is too noticeable—they don't want to be hooked up all the time and worry that it may get in the way of physical activity. Others find it is a constant, unwanted reminder that they have diabetes.
- Some children find that the needle hurts more, because it is a bit bigger than an ordinary insulin needle. On the other hand, there is only one injection every three days. Some

families use anaesthetic cream to numb the site before inserting the cannula.

- The pump is only as good as the person who is running it. Anyone who is using the pump needs to be willing to make decisions and solve problems when they arise.

Concerns for Specific Age Groups

Babies and Toddlers

Babies and toddlers can be good candidates for the pump. Because they are with their parents all the time, the parent can monitor the child easily and react quickly if there are any problems.

Parents may worry that children of this age may push buttons on the pump by accident. Most pumps, however, have a feature that allows parents to "lock out" the child so that only the parents can administer bolus doses.

School-Aged Children

Young school-aged children often cannot check their own blood glucose, calculate bolus doses, or remember to push the button on the pump before meals. But they are away from home during the day, so their parents can't be there to monitor the situation. In Canada (2009), there is highly variable support available at school for children with diabetes. Nonetheless, many families find ways to ensure that their children—those on pumps—get the right kind of support during school hours; discuss the possibilities with the school personnel and members of your diabetes team. For some, e.g., the youngest children, such support might mean that a nurse comes to the school at key intervals during the day to do testing and give insulin; for older children, support from a teacher or other school employee while the child performs the tasks may be all that is required.

Older Children and Teenagers

Preteens and teens are able to check their own blood glucose concentrations and calculate bolus doses. They can take on more of the routine of using the pump. However, it's important for parents to stay involved. One option is to sit down together at the end of the day to review blood glucose readings and bolus doses. Parents and teens can use this time to discuss any problems that came up during the day and work on solving them.

Children in this age group also have more concerns about body image. The pump makes a teen visibly "different," and teens may be uncomfortable about using it in public. Teens who are just starting the pump may also be concerned about gaining weight; if the pump improves glucose control, this in turn will help their bodies use food more efficiently. Weight gain is most likely to occur if blood glucose was poorly controlled before initiating the pump. If this is a concern, the teen should speak with members of the diabetes team in advance and learn ways to minimize the weight gain.

Starting the Insulin Pump

Families who are used to the standard regimen of three insulin injections per day, with rigid planning and counting, need to learn a new way of thinking about diabetes management when they start using the pump. However, most families make this jump successfully.

Before starting to use a pump, make sure you are aware of its advantages and disadvantages. Also check that your diabetes team has experience in the use of pumps among children and teens.

- Different teams start people on pumps in different ways. All will ensure that you and your child have a training session on the technical aspects of the pump. Many teams will use this time to also update your diabetes knowledge and skills including carbohydrate counting. Some programs such as ours at Sick Kids, Toronto, recommend that children and teens wear the pump for a few days with just saline running through it. This allows you to get used to the pump itself; to solve any problems with the tape, the catheter, and the pump; and go through a set change on your own at home. If your child is young, we suggest that he or she starts wearing the waist pack, which will carry the pump, several weeks ahead of time so that your child and classmates can get used to the look and feel of it.

- Next, you will come into the clinic for the actual start. Based on information that you gather with food records and intensive monitoring, members of the team will collaborate with you to calculate and program your basal rates. Similarly, bolus doses and correction factors will be calculated and programmed so that you can use your pump to deliver the right amount of insulin to take care of the carbohydrates in your food and to correct blood glucose levels that are outside of your target. You'll also be advised on how to compensate for exercise.
- You will be asked to call your diabetes nurse or doctor every day, for a short while, to do any problem solving that is required.

As with any system of diabetes management, there is a lot to learn at the beginning, but eventually it gets easier.

Potential Problems When Using the Insulin Pump
Because the pump only provides rapid-acting insulin, blood glucose and ketones can rise very quickly if something goes wrong. It is important to check blood glucose regularly and

address any problems quickly.

The pump is a mechanical device, therefore it can break down. Problems can include:

- batteries running low
- a mechanical problem with the pump
- a clog or a kink in the tubing
- the cannula slipping out of the insertion site
- inflammation or infection at the insertion site, which makes it harder to absorb insulin

A pump has an alarm to alert the wearer when batteries are running low or the tube is clogged. The pump can be set to deliver maximum and minimum bolus rates.

If your child is using an insulin pump, you or your child should always carry:

- a blood glucose meter
- blood glucose test strips
- ketone test strips
- an insulin pen loaded with rapid-acting insulin, in case of pump failure
- a supply of intermediate- or long-acting insulin, if you are going to be somewhere where you will not be able to get a replacement pump within 6–12 hours if your pump malfunctions

Other Devices

There are many devices designed to make injections seem easier; however, none takes away the need for an injection itself. Before investing in any injection aid, talk to your health care team about its usefulness and effectiveness. If your child wants an injection aid to eliminate pain, remind him that all injections hurt a little. If the injection is more painful than usual, try to:

- check the needle—there may be a defect
- insert the needle quickly—slow injections hurt more
- push the plunger in a little more slowly—this will reduce any burning sensation
- keep the insulin out of the refrigerator—children say they can feel cold insulin being injected
- pinch the skin less tightly
- try a different injection site
- avoid using alcohol to clean the injection site, or allow it to dry completely if you do

If none of this works, talk to your diabetes nurse about the selection of injection sites, different kinds of needles, and other tools that may be helpful.

Insertion Aids

For those bothered by inserting a needle, these spring-loaded devices can be useful. With the push of a button, the needle of an insulin-filled syringe is quickly inserted under the skin. Generally, the plunger of the syringe must still be pushed to inject the insulin.

Jet Injectors

Jet injectors are needleless alternatives to syringes. They force insulin through the skin in a high-pressure stream. Although this may seem an ideal way of delivering insulin, injectors are very expensive and require consistent maintenance to keep them sterile. They can cause injury to the skin, such as bruising, and checking the accuracy of the dose can be difficult because some insulin may stay on the surface of the skin. They have not been shown to be less traumatic, physically or emotionally, to the child.

Insuflon

An insuflon is a small Teflon indwelling catheter that is inserted under the skin (similar to a pump site) and taped into place. Insulin is injected with a syringe or pen through the silicon membrane of the insuflon rather than through the skin. The insuflon requires a needle for catheter insertion only once every four or five days.

Insulin Dosages and Frequency

Initially, the diabetes team will determine the insulin dosage and frequency. This is the insulin regimen. It can take a few days to a few weeks of fine-tuning to figure out how much insulin is required. While some children may manage to get excellent blood glucose control on just two or three injections a day in the beginning, eventually most children require a more intensive approach once the honeymoon period is over.

The goal of insulin treatment is to mimic the pancreas in terms of insulin response. Ideally this means that a small amount of insulin is being supplied to the body all of the time (basal insulin) and then extra insulin is given with food or in response to an elevated blood glucose (bolus dose). In the beginning, infants, toddlers, and preschoolers usually receive two injections a day: a mixture of rapid-acting and intermediate- or long-acting insulins before breakfast and again before supper. A change to more frequent injections or the use of an insulin pump is recommended when this basic treatment plan is no longer working to achieve control.

Older children (over 5 or 6 years of age) usually start on three injections a day, using a mix of rapid-acting and intermediate-acting insulin before breakfast, rapid-acting insulin before supper, and intermediate-acting insulin at bedtime. Ideally most teens should move to, and even start on, a multiple-injection-a-day routine, with a dose of rapid-acting insulin before meals and major snacks, and intermediate- or long-acting insulin at bedtime. More injections are not a sign of worsening diabetes. Rather, when used thoughtfully, such a routine allows for a more flexible lifestyle in terms of the timing of meals and sleeping in without compromising excellent control. Furthermore, now that we are convinced of the relationship between blood glucose control and short- and long-term health, there is increased emphasis on doing whatever it takes to achieve healthy blood glucoses. This invariably means more frequent injections or the use of insulin pumps to more closely mimic the pancreas. As your child's situation changes, as we learn more and our tools improve, you should expect changes in the treatment plan.

Remember also that insulin requirements are affected by growth and development, appetite, physical activity, and stress or illness; no fixed dose will work indefinitely. The dose must be adjusted to provide optimal blood glucose control.

In time, as blood glucose levels stabilize and families gain more experience, most parents and teens become quite adept at taking the lead in decisions about adjustments. The diabetes team is always there for advice and backup.

Q&A

I hate needles. How can I expect my 6-year-old to get used to them?

Children take their cues from their parents. Any fear or dislike you have of needles may make your child afraid, too. Some parents find that reminding themselves that the insulin injection allows their child to survive and stay healthy makes injection time easier. If parents say, "I need to give you your insulin so you'll have lots of energy to play and to grow," the child begins to understand, and the parents get over their own apprehension. Follow up each needle with a big hug and kiss, and get on with the day's activities.

My toddler gets a combination of NPH and lispro insulin twice each day. Because the dose is so tiny, it seems I discard the better part of both 10 mL bottles of insulin at the end of each month. Is there any reason I can't use a syringe to withdraw the insulin from a cartridge instead?
Although the insulin manufacturers don't suggest substituting cartridges for bottles, many people find that if they need less than 10 or 15 units of insulin it's less costly to use pen cartridges in place of 10 mL bottles. The unopened cartridges can be stored in the refrigerator until the expiry date, and the open cartridge is discarded after four weeks.

If you use cartridges, don't attempt to put any air into the cartridge before withdrawing the insulin. Simply insert the needle and withdraw the insulin. Inserting air may result in popping out the cork at the other end of the cartridge, in which case the entire cartridge will be ruined. When using NPH insulin do not forget to invert the cartridge twenty times to ensure adequate mixing.

Finally, you may be interested to know that pens with half-unit increments are available on the market, and that these may facilitate the administration of small dosages of insulin in young children.

Our 5-year-old prefers that Mommy give the injections. Is that a problem?
In many families, one person takes on most of the responsibility for injections. Problems arise, however, when that person is unavailable. It's important that all regular caregivers be able to share responsibility for giving the injection, and that the child

feels safe and confident with any of them. Single-parent families should enlist the help of a friend or relative. Some families work out a schedule where one parent takes care of the morning injections and the other parent looks after evening injections.

Sharing the burden is also critical for coping with the daily demands of diabetes and preventing parent burnout.

How old do children have to be before they can give their own injections?
There's no magic age at which children are suddenly capable. Generally, by 9 or 10 years of age, they have the manual dexterity and ability to draw up and give their own insulin. However, children this age lack judgment. Thus they usually require supervision into their teenage years. This means watching your child prepare the dose and insert the needle, checking the expiry date on the insulin bottle and reminding the child to rotate injection sites.

Even at younger ages, many children are curious and want to take part in some aspects of the routine. As they reach the age when they want to go on sleepovers or spend more time away from home, it will become more important for them to show that they can safely manage their own diabetes routines. This is a gradual process for both parents and child. Many children learn to give their first needle or to try new sites at diabetes summer camps.

What if some insulin leaks out of the injection site?
When insulin leaks, don't try to guess the amount lost and replace it. The risk of too much insulin causing a low blood glucose reaction outweighs any benefit. Note it in your logbook and take it into account if the next blood check is high. In the meantime, here are a few tips to minimize such occurrences:

- Get rid of any cause of excess pressure at the injection site, such as a bent leg or a chair pressing against the buttock.
- Gently pinch the skin and pull it slightly to the side before injecting. When you let go, the skin falls back into place and covers the needle track.
- Inject the insulin slowly.
- Let go of the pinched skin before removing the needle to avoid squeezing the insulin back out.
- Count slowly to at least five before removing the needle.
- Apply light pressure on the injection site for a couple of seconds as you remove the needle, to prevent blood and insulin from coming out.
- If you are using a very short needle, try a longer one.

What does it mean if there is bruising at the injection site? This can happen from time to time and it's not harmful. It usually means the needle has nicked a tiny blood vessel. To minimize the chance of bruising, apply gentle pressure to the site with a dry piece of cotton or a clean finger after injecting. Also, be careful not to pinch the skin too tightly or insert the needle too slowly. If you get continuous and excessive bruising, consult your diabetes team.

Are premixed insulins better than mixing your own insulin? Premixed insulins may be more convenient, but they don't give you as much flexibility. With children, the insulin dose changes frequently due to growth and varying appetite and activity. Ideally, families should be able to alter doses of intermediate- and rapid-acting insulins, independent of each other. Premixes don't allow for this.

My son refuses to clean his injection sites with alcohol. Should I be worried?

Most diabetes centers no longer include alcohol swabbing as part of their injection technique. There's no evidence to show that brief alcohol swabbing has any effect when people bathe regularly. Injection-site infections are exceptionally rare.

Why is the injection site all red and itchy?

Some children are sensitive to rubbing alcohol or one of the components of the insulin solution. The redness you see is probably hives—a localized allergic reaction. Changing the brand of insulin may help. In rare cases, someone has an allergic reaction to insulin. Speak to your diabetes team. In most cases the child eventually builds up a tolerance to the insulin and the reaction subsides.

What happens if I accidentally give too much insulin?

Believe it or not, this is not an uncommon mistake. If you've given too much insulin, contact your health care team. You'll need to monitor blood glucose levels every 2 to 3 hours. Set your alarm to wake you up through the night if necessary. You will need to provide extra food to prevent the blood glucose level from falling too low.

What would happen if I accidentally injected an air bubble into my child?

It's not harmful to inject an air bubble under the skin, but if you're injecting air rather than insulin, your child may not be getting the full dose. This will cause a high blood glucose reading.

My son is 12 years of age and has been on the pump for nearly eighteen months. When he first went on the pump his blood glucose concentrations were quite stable and his A1C dropped from 8.4 percent to 6.7 percent. However, during the last six months his A1C has climbed to 8.1 percent and his blood glucose concentrations are all over the place. What is going on and what can I do?

The fact that his A1C dropped to 6.7 percent suggests that pump therapy can work well for your son. However, remember that pump therapy is just another way of giving insulin, it does not measure the blood glucose, and it only gives the amount of insulin that you have programmed it to provide. The primary principles of balancing food, insulin, and exercise remain the same and monitoring of blood glucose before meals and snacks is the guide to this balance.

There are many reasons why your son's blood glucose control may have changed.

- If his diet has changed you must ensure that the pump settings have been changed accordingly.
- If your child has grown or gained weight his pump settings may also require readjusting.
- If his activity has changed, especially if he has gotten into more competitive athletics, his previous pump settings may be giving him too much insulin at some times and not enough at other times. You probably should do more blood glucose testing before, during, and after the activity to provide you with the information to make appropriate changes to the pump settings.
- For insulin to do its job it must be in good shape and get into the body appropriately. Make sure that the insulin in the reservoir is clear, that he is changing his cannula and the

attached catheter frequently enough, and that he is inserting the cannula into smooth and healthy sites.
- The most common reason for deterioration in blood glucose control on a pump is missed boluses. Check the bolus history on the pump and work out a system with your son to remind him to give his insulin at the right times.

In general, just because your son appears comfortable with the pump and its operation does not mean that you should totally back off. Stay in the loop so that you can help him to problem solve.

My 11-year-old daughter has expressed interest in using the pump but is concerned that it may limit her from participating in some of the sports she enjoys so much. Can she still use an insulin pump?

Employing an insulin pump to manage her diabetes should not be an obstacle to her participating in most sports. The key elements to watch out for would be protecting the insertion site, avoiding long exposed lengths of catheter, and securing the pump so that it does not shake free during the sports activities. Some individuals choose specific sites for the catheter insertion which can easily be protected by their sports equipment or outfit. For some activities an extra waistband under the uniform or equipment may successfully be used to secure the pump. Many children disconnect the catheter from the infusion site for periods of about an hour during swim classes or competitions.

FOUR

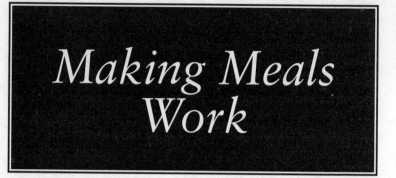

Making Meals Work

Mealtime at Terry and Linda's home is always lively. Both parents like to prepare interesting dishes for their two sons, Michael, 12, and Campbell, 8, who has diabetes. The family's diet is healthy, featuring a variety of foods, even though vegetables are not a favorite. Before being diagnosed with diabetes, Campbell didn't have much of a sweet tooth. However, like most children, he did enjoy the occasional treat.

"I remember when Campbell was diagnosed," recalls Linda. "It was just before his fifth birthday. I was so worried that he wouldn't be allowed to eat any glucose. How were we going to celebrate his birthday without cake and ice cream?" After speaking to the dietitian in the diabetes clinic, Linda realized that they didn't have to make many changes in their eating habits, and that with some planning Campbell could have the cake and ice cream on his birthday.

Even though Campbell has had diabetes for more than three years, Linda and Terry still sometimes find meal planning a challenge. "This winter was Campbell's first year playing hockey," says Terry, noting that early-morning practices, suppertime games, and weekend tournaments present a change from his usual eating routines. But with careful planning, they were able to make the necessary adjustments.

For some families, planning meals is the trickiest part of diabetes management. At first, you look at food very differently than you did before. The simple act of cooking dinner can feel like a science class, with all the measuring and counting. The grocery shopping trips often take much longer than in the past, as nutrition information on food labels gains importance.

As in Terry and Linda's case, many parents ask: Will my child's intake need to be changed?

The answer is that it depends. There are a few important things to consider when planning meals for children and teens with type 1 diabetes. The main goals of feeding a child with diabetes are:

1. to promote normal growth and development
2. to balance the blood glucose levels
3. to satisfy appetite

The meal plan should also be easy to follow, incorporate the child's likes and dislikes, and reflect the family's lifestyle.

The tool most used to measure how many changes need to be made when a child is diagnosed with diabetes is *Canada's Food Guide to Healthy Eating*. For health we all need to eat a variety of foods from the four food groups (grain products, vegetables and fruit, milk products, and meats and alternatives) in certain quantities. This helps ensure that we are getting all our daily vitamins and minerals to keep our bodies healthy. So when you first meet with the dietitian he will make sure that your child is eating the types and amounts of foods that are needed to maintain overall health. If your child already follows the guidelines for healthy eating, it is likely that fewer changes will have to be made.

Canada's Guidelines for Healthy Eating
1. Enjoy a VARIETY of foods
2. Emphasize cereals, breads, other grain products, vegetables, and fruit
3. Choose lower-fat dairy products, leaner meats, and food prepared with little or no fat
4. Achieve and maintain a healthy body weight by enjoying regular physical activity and healthy eating
5. Limit salt, alcohol, and caffeine

Andrea is 7 and is newly diagnosed with diabetes. Let's take a look at her typical food intake before diabetes.

Breakfast   1 bowl of cereal with 2 percent milk

Morning snack   1 cheese stick
(at school)   1 apple

Lunch   1 ham and cheese sandwich on whole wheat bread
                     1 banana
                     1 juice box
                     2 chocolate chip cookies

Afternoon snack   1 granola bar
                     1 yogurt tube

After-school snack 4–5 crackers and cheese
                      1 cup of 2 percent milk

Supper	1 cup of spaghetti with tomato sauce
	green salad with ranch dressing
	milk or water
	occasionally, ice cream for dessert
Bedtime snack	1 piece of toast with peanut butter and
	jam

Looking at Andrea's typical day we see that she is eating a variety of food from all four food groups. She eats many grain products, a variety of vegetables and fruit, some milk and milk products, and some meats and alternatives. These are the first things to consider in order to achieve overall health and to maintain blood glucoses.

It is also important to learn that some foods will raise the blood glucoses while others will not.

How Foods Affect Blood Glucose Level

Ask people what they know about diabetes, and chances are they'll say, "That's the disease where you can't eat sugar, right?" In fact, people with diabetes can and do eat sugar. They simply have to pay close attention to what kinds of sugar and other carbohydrates they eat, how much they eat, and when they eat it. Many foods contain some form of sugar, so learning how much glucose different foods contain is an important aspect of the nutritional management of diabetes. This is called carbohydrate counting. People with diabetes will learn how much insulin they should take for the amount of carbohydrate they are going to eat.

Before thinking about counting carbohydrates we should think about general nutrition. Let's begin with some basic nutrition concepts. The foods we eat provide many nutrients. The three main nutrients, called macronutrients, are protein, fat, and carbohydrate. Vitamins and minerals are micronutrients. Some foods are a combination of protein, fat, and carbohydrate, and therefore appear in all three categories in the food list below.

Carbohydrates
- Starches: breads, pasta, rice, grains, cereals, corn, potatoes, cookies, crackers, roti, dal, legumes
- Fruits and vegetables: all fruits and fruit juices, including tomato juice; sweet vegetables, such as turnip, squash, carrots, peas, beets, parsnip
- Dairy products: milk, yogurt, ice cream, soy beverages
- Glucoses: refined glucose, honey, molasses, syrups, jams and jellies, candy, chocolate, regular soft drinks

Carbohydrates are an essential source of energy. They are important for our muscles, our brains, and our nerves to work properly. Carbohydrate foods are important to consider because they break down into glucose in the body and therefore are the foods that will most rapidly raise blood glucose levels.

There are two types of carbohydrates—simple and complex. Simple carbohydrates are made up of single or paired glucose molecules. They include glucose (also called dextrose), fructose (found in fruits and vegetables), sucrose (found in refined glucose products), and lactose (found in dairy products). When you are reading ingredients labels, note that words ending in "ose" can be classified as glucoses. For example, dextrose and maltose are both glucoses. Complex carbohydrates are made up of many glucose molecules linked together. Complex carbohydrates are found in starch-based foods such as cereal, bread, pasta, rice, and potato.

We used to think that all simple carbohydrates raised the blood glucose quickly while complex carbohydrates raised the blood glucose level slowly; however we now know that this is not true. Generally, foods that contain more refined carbohydrates (simple or complex) or concentrated forms of carbohydrates will raise the blood glucose quickly. Examples of refined carbohydrates include white flour, white bread, and baked goods such as donuts and cookies. Concentrated carbohydrates such as candies, chocolate, regular soft drinks, honey, corn syrup, and liquid invert glucose are other common sweeteners that contain simple carbohydrates and raise blood glucose levels rapidly. The simple glucoses found in milk and milk products, and fruits and vegetables, are slow to absorb into the blood because of all the other nutrients in these foods.

The glycemic index (GI) is a ranking system that compares how fast the carbohydrate-containing foods will raise the blood glucose compared to plain glucose. Foods that raise the blood glucose slower than glucose are said to have a low GI and foods that raise the blood glucose faster than glucose are said to have a high GI. There is also a category for foods that are neither fast nor slow and this is called medium GI. Generally foods that have a low GI are less processed and higher in fiber (e.g., whole grain breads and cereals, oats and oat products, whole fruits and vegetables, legumes, and milk). Foods that have a high GI are more refined and have less fiber, such as white breads and refined cereals (cornflakes and sugary cereals). Children with diabetes should try to include more foods that fall into the low glycemic index categories to help prevent a quick rise in blood glucose and maintain a healthy blood glucose balance.

That is not to say that youngsters with diabetes will never be able to eat glucose and foods containing added glucose, such as candy and chocolate. These foods are fine in moderation—up to 10 percent of their total calorie intake. Learning how to incorporate such foods into the diet is an important part of managing diabetes.

Protein
- Meat, poultry, fish, shellfish
- Eggs
- Milk, cheese, cottage cheese, and other dairy products
- Legumes (nuts, beans and lentils, peanuts and peanut butter, tofu)

With the exception of milk, yogurt, ice cream, and legumes (which also contain carbohydrate), protein foods do not directly raise blood glucose levels. During prolonged starvation or undernutrition however, the body can break protein down into glucose. On a daily basis proteins are essential for growth and to promote healing and tissue repair. Protein foods also provide essential vitamins and minerals.

Fats
- All oils: lard, shortening, margarine
- Meat: especially red meat, but also fowl
- Fish and shellfish
- Dairy products: butter, milk, cream and cream products, cheese and cheese products
- Eggs
- Other: salad dressings (low fat and regular), gravies, nuts, seeds, olives, coconut, avocado

Fats are the major component of such foods as butter, margarine, oil, most salad dressings, and gravies. Often people think that when a person has diabetes she needs to limit her intake of dietary fat quite drastically. However, like proteins, fats do not directly raise the level of blood glucose. Fats are an important part of a well-balanced diet because they also provide essential building blocks for growth and development. So children with diabetes do not need to cut the fat from their diet completely, but should eat higher-fat foods in moderation for overall health and heart health.

There are three types of fats:

- Saturated fats are usually solid at room temperature and tend to raise blood cholesterol. They are found in butter, lard, and shortening, and animal products, such as meat, eggs, and milk. Trans fats have gained a lot of public attention in the past few years. This type of fat is found in baked goods, such as cookies, muffins, and French fries. Trans fats act the same way in the body as saturated fats, by raising blood cholesterol, and therefore their intake should be limited.
- Polyunsaturated fats, which are found in vegetable oils, such as safflower, sunflower, corn, and soybean, sesame, and most nut oils, are usually liquid at room temperature. Nuts and seeds, or soft margarines made with these oils, tend to be associated with lower blood cholesterol.
- Monounsaturated fats are found in other oils, including olive, peanut, and canola, as well as soft margarine made from these oils. These fats may lower blood cholesterol levels if used in place of saturated fats.

These three types of fats are found in varying combinations in foods. It is wise to try to limit the amount of fat in the diet of people more than two years of age, and to try to choose foods that contain polyunsaturated or monounsaturated fats. Maintaining normal lipid (blood fat) levels is important, as high levels contribute to the risk of developing certain complications later in life.

Free Foods
Some vegetables—lettuce, celery, cucumbers, and peppers, for example—fall outside the three categories of carbohydrates, proteins, and fats. They are essential, however, because they add vitamins, minerals, and fiber to the diet, as well as flavor and variety. Since they don't contain macronutrients, they can be considered "free" foods.

Will My Child Need to Follow a Diabetic Diet?
The term "diabetic diet" was used many years ago and referred to a way of eating that someone with diabetes needed to follow. As you have already read, the diabetes way of eating is based on the same guidelines as those for the rest of the population. Today, we tend not to use that term or that method but instead work out a healthy way of eating to achieve optimal blood glucose levels as well as other health goals.

There are two different meal-planning systems that can be used to achieve these targets. Families of school-aged children (5–12 years) are often taught a meal plan and encouraged to keep foods consistent from day to day. Families of older children (teens and pre-teens) are taught a more flexible meal-planning system that focuses on using insulin to carbohydrate (CHO) ratios, which allow for flexibility rather than consistency. Both systems are based on the concept mentioned earlier: carbohydrate counting. Meal planning for infants and toddlers will be discussed separately, later in the chapter.

What Is Carbohydrate Counting?
Now that you know which foods contain carbohydrate, it is

important to start thinking about how much carbohydrate is in each of the foods that your child eats.

The Canadian Diabetes Association's (CDA) meal planning guide, *Beyond the Basics: Meal Planning for Diabetes Prevention and Management*, is a useful tool for learning how to count carbohydrates. Some people may be familiar with the CDA's former meal planning system called the *Good Health Eating Guide*. This has been recently revised to match the meal planning systems found in other countries. *Beyond the Basics* divides all foods into seven categories; grains and starches, fruits, milk and alternatives, vegetables, meat and alternatives, fats, and other choices. All the carbohydrate-containing foods are listed in the servings (or carbohydrate choices) that will provide 15 grams of carbohydrate. The table below shows the carbohydrate content of some common foods.

Beyond the Basics lists all vegetables together, however certain vegetables contain enough carbohydrate to raise blood glucose. Carrots, peas, turnip, squash, beets, and parsnips are the sweeter vegetables that need to be considered with the carbohydrate-

Carbohydrate Content of Some Common Foods

Starch 15 grams	Fruits 15 grams	Milk 15 grams	Snacks & Glucoses 15 grams
• 1 slice of bread	• 1 medium apple, orange, banana, pear	• 1 cup (250 mL) of milk	• 3 cups (750 mL) of popcorn
• ½ cup (125 mL) of pasta		• ½ cup (125 mL) chocolate milk	• 3 digestive cookies
• 1/3 cup (75 mL) of rice	• ½ cup (125 mL) of juice	• 1 small container of yogurt	• 3 teaspoons (15 mL) of sugar
• ½ medium potato			
• 1 6-inch (15-cm) chapati			

Nutrition Facts	
Per container (175 g)	

Amount	% Daily Value
Calories 170	
Fat 4.5 g	7 %
Saturated Fat 3.5 g + Trans Fat 0 g	18 %
Cholesterol 10 mg	
Sodium 85 mg	4 %
Carbohydrate 27 g	9 %
Fibre 0 g	0 %
Sugars 26 g	
Protein 6 g	

Vitamin A	15 %	Vitamin C	0 %
Calcium	20 %	Iron	0 %

containing foods. For one half cup (125 mL) serving, each of these vegetables provides about 10 grams of carbohydrate.

Nutrition facts on pre-packaged foods will provide information on carbohydrate content. Your dietitian will teach you how to read a Nutrition Facts panel.

Meal Planning for School-Aged Children

Stephen was 7 years old when he was diagnosed with diabetes. Although he was a very dependable young boy, he was too young to take the sole responsibility of injecting insulin. In collaboration with the diabetes team, Stephen's parents determined that the best way to control his blood glucoses was by using a routine that required a combination of intermediate- and rapid-acting insulin and an insulin injection three times a day (at breakfast, suppertime, and bedtime). The crucial element of this routine is that once insulin has been injected, it can't be "turned off." Therefore, a steady supply of glucose, in the form of carbohydrate, must be provided to maintain blood glucose balance and avoid excessive levels (low or high) of blood glucoses. The type of meal plan developed for Stephen consisted of three main meals and two to four snacks each day.

The goal is to have a consistent amount of carbohydrate at the same time each day, thereby making it easier to determine the appropriate insulin dose. It was important that the amount of food both satisfied Stephen's appetite and provided enough nutrients for proper growth. Consistency is the key to successful meal planning on this insulin regime. However, any meal plan should be flexible and realistic, and must take into account the individual's lifestyle, likes, and dislikes.

The dietitian will likely encourage you to record your child's food intake for three days. Based on these records, the dietitian will help you plan a certain amount of carbohydrate and will encourage you to choose foods from each group for the child's meals and snacks. This system will become easy to apply, with some instruction from your dietitian and practice using available lists.

Now that Stephen's normal appetite has returned, the dietitian has provided him and his parents with a meal plan. Here's a look at what Stephen eats during the day and the amount of carbohydrate these quantities represent.

Figure 4: A 24-Hour Record of Stephen's Food Consumption

Meal	Food consumed	Amount of carbohydrate
Breakfast	1 slice of toast	15 g
	butter	0 g
	1 tsp (5 ml) of jam	2 g
	1 cup (250 mL) of milk	15 g
Morning snack	1 granola bar	15 g
Lunch	1 tuna salad sandwich	30 g
	1 drinkable yogurt	10 g

	2 cookies	15 g
	1/2 apple	7.5 g
Afternoon snack	1 pear	15 g
Supper	1/2 potato	15 g
	1 chicken drumstick	0 g
	1 stalk of broccoli	0 g
	1/4 cup (60 mL) of carrots	5 g
	1 cup (250 mL) of milk	15 g
Evening snack	1/2 cup (125 mL) of cereal	15 g
	1/2 cup (125 mL) of milk	7.5 g

Stephen's parents and the dietitian determine that this is a very usual intake for Stephen, so the dietitian encouraged Stephen's parents to stick to the following amounts of carbohydrate on a daily basis:

Plan
Breakfast: 30 g
Morning snack: 15 g
Lunch: 60 g
Afternoon snack: 15 g
Supper: 35 g
Evening snack: 20 g

Tonight the family is having spaghetti and meat sauce, salad, rolls, and strawberries for dessert. Stephen's meal plan calls for supper to consist of 35 grams of carbohydrate. So Stephen can have:

1/2 cup (125 mL) spaghetti: 15 g
1 small dinner roll: 15 g
1 cup (250 mL) strawberries: 7.5 g
Water
Total carbohydrate = 37.5 g

You can see that in order to allow Stephen the flexibility of having the amount of spaghetti that he would like, we substituted his usual drink of milk (from the food records) and suggested water to maintain consistency in carbohydrate. He can also have the meat sauce and the salad to provide him with some protein and vegetable. We don't need to count the amount of protein, fats, or vegetables at this point as Stephen's diet appears well rounded and his growth is normal.

The Importance of Consistency

Satisfaction with the Amount of Food Is Important

Remember that a meal plan is not a diet in the sense of limiting food. It's important for children to feel satisfied, so their meal plans will change as they grow. Children and parents need to be aware when and if hunger increases. The dietitian will help parents adjust the meal plan to allow more food, and the doctor or diabetes nurse will adjust a child's insulin dosage to balance the effect of the extra food on his or her blood glucose.

At the outset of diabetes, it is important for all children and teens to be as consistent as possible (from day to day) in the timing, amounts, and types of food eaten during snacks and meals. This will help them achieve and maintain the best possible control over their blood glucose. If, for example, a 12-year-old boy eats an enormous dinner one night but skips dinner the next, it makes the task of adjusting his insulin dose and preventing high and low blood glucose reactions very difficult. Those using rapid- or short-acting insulin before each meal, and those using insulin pumps, will quickly develop more flexibility in the timing and amount of food they eat, but they too need a period of consistency at the beginning, to work out their insulin to carbohydrate ratio—that is, the amount of carbohydrate they can metabolize with 1 unit of insulin. One unit of insulin usually metabolizes 5 to 20 grams of carbohydrate, but the ratio varies from one person to another.

In time, most young people and their families learn to be more flexible about their meal plans; for example, they may choose a different dose of rapid-acting insulin before a meal, based on the meal's expected carbohydrate content. Some will even give more insulin after a meal if more carbohydrate has been ingested.

Knowing that mealtimes and the amounts of food eaten are consistent also helps rule out food as the cause of high or low blood glucose readings. For example, a new after-school activity is planned. The extra exercise will likely cause a lower blood glucose reading. If the child has swayed from the meal plan, and perhaps also skipped a snack, the parents can't be sure of the real cause of the low blood glucose.

Joey arrives home from school earlier than expected because his soccer practice is canceled. He usually has his snack before practice at 3:30 p.m., but since he doesn't have practice today, and he's not really that hungry, he decides to skip it. By 4:00 p.m., however, he is feeling hungry, so he eats his snack then. When he checks his blood glucose at 5:30 p.m., it's a little high. Is it high because he didn't burn off the energy he usually consumes during soccer practice, or because he had his snack later than usual and didn't have two hours between eating and testing his blood glucose?

While not every high or low blood glucose reading can or should be accounted for, understanding the relationships between food, insulin, and activity is important to help you determine whether an insulin adjustment is necessary. While it is tempting to try to correct low or high readings by overeating or withholding food, this can lead to a lot of confusion. For example, let's look at Joey again. His 5:30 p.m. reading is high, so he eats less dinner in order to bring down his blood glucose level. Before bed, he's a little low so he eats a few extra cookies. He gets up twice that night to go to the bathroom and wakes up with a high reading. To avoid increasing his blood glucose further, he eats only half a bowl of cereal instead of a whole bowlful. By morning recess he starts to feel faint and nauseated with a low blood glucose reaction. This roller coaster is known as "chasing blood glucoses." It can be frustrating and potentially dangerous.

What Is the Meal Planning System for Older Children?

Multiple Daily Injections and Carbohydrate Counting

Adam is a 14-year-old boy who was diagnosed with type 1 diabetes last year. He is extremely active, playing hockey several times a week in the winter and soccer in the summer. His family eats meals at times that fit with game and practice times. This often means that supper ranges from as early as 4 p.m. to as late as 9 p.m. Because consistency with meal times was a real challenge for Adam, he and his parents decided on a flexible insulin routine that would allow for the flexible meal and snack times that his activities required—without compromising the excellent control he wanted and needed for good performance.

As you have already read, one of the most effective ways to manage diabetes is by a multiple daily injection routine. Teens who follow this routine will take a long-acting insulin once or twice a day and rapid-acting insulin with their meals and some snacks. The benefits of this routine are that the child can eat what and when he wants, and inject the amount of insulin needed for the carbohydrate consumed. The insulin to carbohydrate ratio (CHO) is used to determine the insulin dose that the child takes pre-meal. It refers to the number of units of insulin required to metabolize each gram of carbohydrate in the meal. So it is important on this system to learn carbohydrate counting very well. In Adam's case, he would count up the carbohydrate in his supper and give a calculated dose depending on his estimated intake. When hockey games are early, he will eat dinner early so that he has the fuel necessary for the game.

Adam can also vary the amount of carbohydrate that he feels like eating. For example, the diabetes team may have determined that Adam needs 1 unit of rapid-acting insulin for every 10 grams of carbohydrate. Let's say that he is eating the following meal for supper:

Stir fry with 2 cups (500 mL) of rice: 90 g
1 cup (250 mL) of milk: 12 g
Total: 102 g

For 102 g of carbohydrate he would need 10 units of insulin.
Occasionally Adam goes out for pizza with friends:

4 slices of pizza: 120 g
Diet coke   0 g
Total   120 g

Adam would need 12 units of fast-acting insulin for this meal. So even though he is not being consistent about how much carbohydrate he eats, Adam is being consistent with the ratio of insulin to carbohydrate that he needs and injects the correct amount when he is eating. This allows him the freedom to eat many different types of meals and still keep his blood glucoses in target. In addition, using this system he is able to correct for glucose levels outside of his target range before meals.

Meal Planning for the Infant or Toddler

Infants and toddlers experience daily fluctuations in appetite, making it difficult to stick to a meal plan. One day they may have a spoonful of cereal for breakfast, nibble at a sandwich for lunch, and have a tiny piece of meat for supper. The next day, they might eat an entire bowl of cereal to start the day, milk and cookies for snacks, a peanut butter sandwich and banana for lunch, and chicken and potatoes for supper. Young children may go through periods when they want to eat the same thing every day, followed by periods when they refuse to touch their previous favorites.

It is neither practical nor realistic to set up a strict meal plan for a young child with diabetes. Rather, meal planning should focus on normal infant or toddler feeding, emphasizing healthy eating and a variety of foods during the day, as well as consistency in the timing of meals and snacks and avoiding an excessive amount of simple glucoses, such as juices. Furthermore, because of the unpredictable eating patterns of young children, and their inability to communicate hypoglycemia, their pre-meal blood glucose goals will be higher than those of older children (6–12 mmol/L or 110–220 mg/dL).

As children grow older, the approach to meal planning should be changed to incorporate the principles of carbohydrate counting and a consistent meal plan appropriate for age. This often occurs when the child starts spending more time in a school setting, such as the transition from kindergarten to first grade. In the meantime, it is certainly helpful for parents to learn the carbohydrate content of different foods, for two reasons. It allows them to offer a consistent amount of carbohydrate from day to day; and if the child is receiving a dose of rapid-acting insulin with the meal, it allows the parents to adjust the dose to the amount of carbohydrate actually eaten.

Some families will choose to follow an MDI routine for their toddlers. In this case they will count the carbohydrate that they think the child will eat and give insulin based on an insulin to carbohydrate ratio. Some will also choose to give the rapid-acting insulin immediately following the meal so that they are better able to match the insulin with the carbohydrate eaten.

Eating Out

Fast Food

Diabetes doesn't mean that families can no longer enjoy the convenience of "fast food." Here are some exchange guidelines for common fast food fare:

- I hamburger = 2 starch, 2 protein, 2 fat = 30 g
- I small fries (about 20) = 2 starch, 2 fat = 30 g
- I slice medium cheese pizza = 2 starch, 2 protein, 2 fat = 30 g
- 6-inch (15 cm) sub sandwich = 3 starch, 2 protein, 2 fat = 45 g

Most fast-food chains can supply exchange guidelines for their menus, on request.

For the first few weeks after diagnosis, parents may be nervous about taking their child out for dinner. However, many fast-food restaurants will supply nutritional information about their dishes on request. This information may also be found online. As well, parents shouldn't feel shy about explaining to waiters that someone in the family has diabetes and that if the meal will be delayed they need to know. In this event, nibbling on a breadstick or some crackers until the meal arrives is a good strategy, but these should be included as part of the meal's carbohydrates. Rapid-acting insulin is a major advantage for eating out, because the injection can be given when the meal is served, with the dose adjusted to the meal's carbohydrate content.

Friends who don't know much about diabetes may be worried about what to feed the child. It helps to take the lead and invite friends over first so they can see that Joey still eats hot dogs, just as he used to. When eating at a friend's house, ask what time they intend to serve dinner and provide some guidance. Children may be able to switch their bedtime snack and dinner if dinner is being served much later than usual.

Q&A

Can my child have birthday cake again?
Yes. In fact, many children are so excited with the party's fun and games that the food stays on the plate. The key is to ensure that the adult in charge is aware that the child needs to eat something. And if the blood glucose is high that evening, note the reason in your child's logbook, and move on.

What about Halloween?
Halloween is a special time of year for many children and parents alike. Children with diabetes shouldn't be deprived of the chance to dress up and parade around the neighborhood in search of treats. Treats can be monitored and worked into the meal plan. Remember that Halloween night's extra activity should be planned for with extra food—perhaps one small

chocolate bar for each 20 to 30 minutes out on the streets. The remaining treats can be part of a meal or snack or can be used as extra food for planned activities. Remember how you handled Halloween candy before your child had diabetes, and try not to make too much of it. Trade some of the lollipops, candy, and regular gum for chips, sugar-free gum, or even a trip to the movies. Be creative!

People keep telling me that lentils and beans are good for people with diabetes. Should I introduce these into my family's diet?
Lentils and beans are excellent sources of low-fat protein and are commonly suggested for people with type 2 diabetes. If you already prepare dishes using these foods, that's fine. Do not feel, however, that you should make radical changes in the foods your family eats. Adjusting to diabetes is difficult enough! If you want to introduce new foods to your table, wait until you have the other aspects of diabetes management—blood glucose testing, insulin injections, and the meal plan—under control. Some legumes produce bloating and gas, so go slowly if these are not a usual part of your family's diet.

My 3-year-old wants to eat only macaroni. Is this normal?
Many younger children have a limited number of foods they like to eat. However, children—especially toddlers—will decide on a whim that what was the *only* food choice for three weeks is now totally unacceptable. With a child with diabetes, be ready to offer other appealing options. Foods such as cereal or a grilled cheese sandwich are good choices. Keep food fun by arranging servings in a unique way, or cutting food into interesting shapes. Children love to dip anything—vegetables into dip, crackers into soup. They may also respond to food more readily if they are involved in the selection. Ask what they want

from the grocery store, or have them help fill the cart. You can even involve them in preparing the dish in a safe, appropriate way, such as arranging chopped vegetables in a dish.

My toddler sometimes decides he doesn't want to eat—after I've already given the insulin. Should I force him to eat?
Forcing a child to eat usually leaves both the parents and the child upset and frustrated. Toddlers will usually take juice or milk, both sources of carbohydrate, so taking the meal away and offering either milk or juice is an appropriate thing to do. Watch carefully for a low blood glucose reaction and treat it appropriately. They'll probably be hungry for their next meal or snack, since they ate little or nothing earlier. If food refusal happens often, talk to your diabetes team. You may need to reduce the insulin and adjust the blood glucose targets. Or ask your doctor about giving the insulin injection immediately after the meal, and adjusting the dose to the amount of carbohydrate eaten.

Is it safe to eat a vegetarian diet with diabetes?
A vegetarian diet is safe for people with diabetes, provided all nutritional needs are being met, as in people without diabetes. Your dietitian will be a great source of information and support as you strive to make healthy choices.

What about fasting—can people with diabetes participate in rituals of Ramadan or Yom Kippur?
Fasting can be dangerous for anyone who takes insulin. Generally, people with diabetes are exempt from these rituals, but check with the appropriate religious authority. In many cases, specific guidelines have been developed. Older children and teenagers using an insulin pump or a multiple daily insulin

routine with a long-acting basal insulin and rapid-acting insulin with meals will be able to fast more safely as the basal insulin will allow for blood glucose control during time without food, without increasing the risk of hypoglycemia.

Do I really need to start measuring all these portions?
It may seem inconvenient at first, but measuring food will help you learn to estimate portion sizes. After a while, you won't need to double-check every measurement. However, it's a good idea to go back to measuring foods from time to time, to be sure that your estimates are still fairly accurate.

I'm going crazy counting carbohydrates. I'm worried about making a mistake.
Initially, many parents are overwhelmed by the amount of planning and measuring involved in following a meal plan, and start to plan their meals according to the number of carbohydrates suggested. Instead, it's easier to plan meals as you usually would, and then look at the carbohydrate count and give appropriate portions to make up the amount that your child's meal plan states. Remember to include food from all food groups—grains and cereals, fruits and vegetables, meats and alternates, and dairy products—and you'll be providing a balanced diet that meets the requirements of diabetes.

Should I put my child on a low-fat diet, or can we still eat burgers and fries occasionally?
Fat is an important part of a growing child's diet, and you should resist eliminating it from the diet altogether. However, we don't generally have to go out of our way to work fat into the North American child's diet. The occasional meal of burgers and fries can be part of a healthy diet as long as this is an occasional treat and high-fat meals are not eaten regularly.

My child puts ketchup on everything. Is the glucose in ketchup going to affect his blood glucose?

The small amount of glucose (3 grams or less in 2 tsp/10 mL) found in reasonable serving sizes of ketchup, barbecue sauce, store-bought salad dressings, or peanut butter is not enough to elevate blood glucose levels significantly.

Is it safe to use glucose substitutes?

The sweeteners commonly found in grocery stores (also found in diet foods and diet drinks) have been approved by the government. For most of these products the government has set an acceptable daily intake (ADI), which is the average amount people can use every day of their lives without risk of harm. The ADI is based on body weight, but there's a very large safety margin. The dietitian on your team can give you specific information about particular sweeteners.

It's worth noting that certain sweeteners, such as sorbitol (often found in gum and dietetic candy), may cause some diarrhea.

FIVE

Balancing Blood Glucose

Twelve-year-old Jason isn't very athletic, but he loves a snowy winter evening—especially when it's not a school night. Often, on a Friday night after dinner, he and his friends head off to the local toboggan hill for a couple of hours of slipping and sliding. Jason has diabetes, but he has no trouble keeping up with his tobogganing buddies. He can easily match them run for run. In fact, he can even join them for a nice big mug of hot chocolate with marshmallows at the end of the evening. Jason has learned he can do almost anything his friends can do, with a little planning.

Jason knows that walking up the toboggan hill will use up a lot of energy. If he takes his usual amount of insulin and eats the usual amount of food, his blood glucose will go low—probably when he's out on the hill. He also knows that he can't pass up the hot chocolate on these nights—after all, tobogganing and hot chocolate go hand in hand. So he and his parents agree on a slight reduction in the suppertime rapid-acting insulin, a mug of hot chocolate after tobogganing, and a blood glucose test before bed. Even though hot chocolate is a higher-glucose bedtime snack than usual, the extra activity after dinner means Jason can afford the extra carbohydrate.

As parents and child or teen continue to learn more about diabetes, they begin to feel more confident about the decisions they are making. Children become accustomed to checking their blood glucose level four or more times a day; parents are less nervous about giving insulin injections; older children start to recognize the feelings they get when their blood glucose starts to fall. Parents consult their diabetes team less often, primarily because they now know the answers to a lot of their own questions and are better able to deal with new situations. By including children in the discussion and problem solving, they can pave the way for future independence.

Why Monitor?

Blood glucose monitoring is an essential part of evaluating the blood glucose balance and diabetes control. Blood glucose results provide valuable information about when to adjust the dose and by how much. As children grow they need more insulin. And there are other factors that may make the blood glucose go high or low temporarily such as activity level, illness, extra food, and so on. Blood glucose checks provide the information needed to allow you to correct out-of-range glucoses and achieve safe and healthy blood glucose control.

Other monitoring tools that we'll discuss in this chapter include urine testing for glucose and ketones, and a blood test for glycosylated (or glycated) hemoglobin—A1C—each of which reflects diabetes control during the previous three-month period.

Your diabetes team will help you become familiar with each of these tools. It is important to remember that such checks are useful only when they are done accurately and interpreted wisely.

Setting the Blood Glucose Target Range

The blood glucose targets change at various stages of growth and development. Target ranges are defined by the child's and parents' or other caregiver's ability to understand diabetes, interpret signs and feelings of low blood glucose levels, and

Blood Glucose Target Ranges

Age	Characteristic/ability	Acceptable target range (before meals)
infants/toddlers/ preschoolers	• unable to recognize or communicate signs and symptoms of low blood glucose reaction • unpredictable eating	6–12 mmol/L (110–220 mg/dL)
school-age children and some young adolescents	• able to recognize or communicate signs and symptoms of low blood glucose reaction • more predictable eating • somewhat lacking in judgment • reliant on others for adjusting treatment and planning ahead	4–10 mmol/L (70–180 mg/dL)
most adolescents and young adults	• able to recognize and treat low blood glucose reactions • understand concept of balance • capable of predictable eating —for those on insulin pumps, the range may be 4–7 mmol/L (70–125 mg/dL) before meals and below 9 mmol/L (160 mg/dL) after • able to plan ahead	4–8 mmol/L (70–145 mg/dL)

act on them. They are negotiated with the diabetes team, all of whom should have the same goals.

When to Check Blood Glucose

For children and teens receiving two to four insulin injections daily, checking blood glucose levels before each meal and before the bedtime snack tells you how the insulin is working. But one test cannot tell the whole story. Each test gives a unique and important piece of information.

In general, testing is performed before meals and provides useful information to guide insulin dose adjustment and correction. In addition, it may be recommended that, from time to time, blood glucose levels be checked 90–120 minutes after a meal. This provides information about how well the insulin is matching the mealtime carbohydrate content and whether the pre-meal dose of rapid-acting insulin is working well enough. Glucose testing four times a day (before each meal and before the bedtime snack) is ideal but may be a challenge. For example, a lunchtime check in young children in daycare or school may be difficult, and the support and willingness of the staff will be needed. Older school-age children may also find lunchtime tests inconvenient, but they should be encouraged to do them. Parents and the rest of the diabetes team should work to help reduce the barriers to lunchtime checking. In addition, an occasional check in the middle of the night helps detect those at risk for late-night lows.

Sometimes blood glucose should be checked apart from the routine—for example, before, during, or after a vigorous activity such as a dance class or football practice, to determine how that particular activity affects the child's glucose level, or during illness or other times of stress.

If the blood glucose is consistently outside the target range (too low or too high), at least four daily checks are needed to determine the appropriate insulin dose adjustment. It is also useful to check between midnight and four in the morning as this is often the lowest time of the day.

Additional testing should also be done:

- if symptoms of low blood glucose are present
- at least every 4 hours during an illness
- at other times prescribed by the diabetes team, or when you're trying to problem-solve or gather information about the impact of a certain food or activity

It is important that children and teens using insulin pumps check their blood glucose more frequently to detect pump problems before symptoms develop and to maximize the benefits of pump therapy.

How to Check Blood Glucose

Since about 1980 it has been possible for people with diabetes to check their blood glucose levels at home. While blood glucose monitoring at home may not be quite as precise as laboratory methods, it is certainly accurate enough for the daily management of diabetes. Home glucose monitoring is performed with a blood glucose meter. Meters require a drop of blood from a finger prick or, for some newer meters, from an alternate site such as the forearm or thigh.

The blood sample is placed on a small area on a special test strip. A chemical in the strip reacts with the glucose in the drop of blood and a small electrical current is produced. The size of the current depends on the blood glucose level. The current is then displayed on the screen of the meter as a blood glucose concentration. Blood glucose meters provide accurate, quick

Lancing device and meter

meter

lancing device

readings of blood glucose when used correctly.

Lancing devices are spring-loaded tools that, at the touch of a button, activate a lancet to prick the finger to obtain a drop of blood. The actual lancet is a small plastic insert with a very short needletip end. The tips come in different sizes, or gauges. The higher the gauge, the finer the point, which helps to get a blood sample less painfully. In addition, some of the lancing devices make it possible to adjust the depth of the finger prick, which further reduces the pain. Even young children may be able to take their own blood samples, with adult supervision. To avoid spreading infections, your lancing device should not be shared with anyone else.

Choosing a Blood Glucose Meter

When you obtain a glucose meter, there are a number of factors to consider. Most important, does your diabetes team have confidence in the accuracy of this meter? Other possible factors are:

- the size of the meter and whether it's easy to take to school, to work, or to the gym
- the time required to perform a blood test
- how much blood is required to get a reliable test result
- how easy it is to operate
- what error messages you get if there is a problem with the test strip or the technique
- how easy it is to calibrate the meter
- whether the meter has memory capacity
- whether it can be downloaded to a computer

Whichever meter you prefer, consider how firmly the manufacturer stands behind its product. Does it provide a toll-free number for questions and technical support?

Most glucose meters come as a kit that includes a finger-pricking or lancing device, a few check strips, control solution, and a carrying case.

Ensuring Accuracy
To ensure that the glucose meter is working properly, it should be checked regularly with the check strips and control solution supplied with the system. At every clinic visit, if possible—and at least once or twice a year—a blood glucose test should be done on the same sample, both in the lab and by your meter to check its accuracy. Results of the meter test should be within 10 to 15 percent of the lab test. For example, if the lab reading is 10.0 mmol/L (180 mg/dL), the meter result should be between 8.5 and 11.5 mmol/L (150–210 mg/dL).

Checking Urine

For Glucose

Because blood glucose checks are now the primary method of assessing diabetes control at home, urinary glucose is usually checked only as a backup to checking blood glucose, or to screen other family members. A chemically treated strip is dipped briefly into a fresh urine sample. As with blood glucose checks, the strip will change color. After a defined period of time the strip is compared with a color chart on the box.

A urine check showing no glucose indicates that when the urine was formed the blood glucose level was below the renal threshold (about 8.0–12.0 mmol/L, or 145–220 mg/dL). If the urine shows glucose, the blood glucose was above the threshold when the urine was formed. These urine checks are at best an indirect measure of blood glucose, because the urine collected for the test may have been produced over a number of hours.

Checking urine for glucose is most useful as a screening tool for other members of the family, if they show signs of diabetes, such as frequent and excessive urination. People without diabetes should expect to find no glucose in the urine. If the urine check shows glucose in someone without diabetes further tests at the doctor's office are required to rule out diabetes. These should be done immediately.

For Ketones

Urinary ketones are tested by dipping a chemically treated strip in a fresh sample of urine, and comparing the color change to a chart. A purple color indicates ketones in the urine. Ketones are a sign of excessive breakdown of fat in the body. This can have a number of causes, including too little insulin or the stress of an illness. They may be detected in someone who doesn't have diabetes if the person is starving or dieting to excess. In that case, though, the blood glucose level should be normal or low, rather than high. Ketones are a cause for concern if they are present when the blood glucose is high (greater than 14 mmol/L or 250 mg/dL).

Check urine ketones whenever:

- blood glucose level is over 14 mmol/L (250 mg/dL) for three readings in a row
- the child is feeling ill, has a fever, or has vomited
- the child has symptoms of high blood glucose, e.g., increased thirst and urination
- the diabetes team asks you to check for ketones—perhaps when the insulin dose is being adjusted

Have strips at home for ketone testing at all times. Ensure that the expiration date on the bottle has not passed and that the bottle is kept closed. Once the bottle is open, the strips must be used within six months.

Note that strips are available to check for ketones and glucose at the same time. Follow the instructions on the package carefully, and ask your health care team for help if the instructions are not clear.

Checking Blood Ketones

More recently it has become possible to check blood ketones at home as an alternative to urine ketone checking. Blood ketone checks may be particularly useful for young children who are unable to void on demand and children and teens using insulin pump therapy. A special meter capable of measuring blood ketones is required for this purpose.

Record-Keeping

The first step in spotting trends in glucose levels is to set up a logbook and complete it daily. Effective diabetes management is like putting the pieces of a puzzle together, and you can't complete the puzzle without all the pieces. Many pharmacies and pharmaceutical companies provide logbooks specially designed for diabetes management. Children can also make their own. A logbook should document:

- the amount and timing of each insulin injection
- the time and result of each blood glucose check
- the results of any urine tests for ketones
- any unusual circumstances related to the diabetes (e.g., a missed snack, a minor illness or strenuous activity, and all insulin reactions—including the time of day and, if possible, the cause of the reaction)

Why all the effort? Accurate daily records will help parents, the child, and the team decide when changes are needed in the insulin dose or meal plan. Be sure to immediately record the results of tests and the amounts of insulin given. These numbers are difficult to remember or to figure out after several days have gone by.

Children need help recording these measurements at first, but as they get older they should be able to maintain their own logbook. Parents should check the book regularly to stay informed, and to make sure the child is recording daily measurements diligently and accurately. Record-keeping can be tedious, so don't be surprised if the child needs help from time to time.

A number of glucose meters have memory to store the time and result of a given blood glucose check. As a result, it's tempting not to record results right away because "it's all in the meter." This can be a problem. Although the meter's memory capabilities may mean that you don't have to download results into the logbook as often, the meter doesn't replace the logbook. Without a well-kept record, it is almost impossible to recognize patterns of blood glucose levels and to make appropriate adjustments in a timely way.

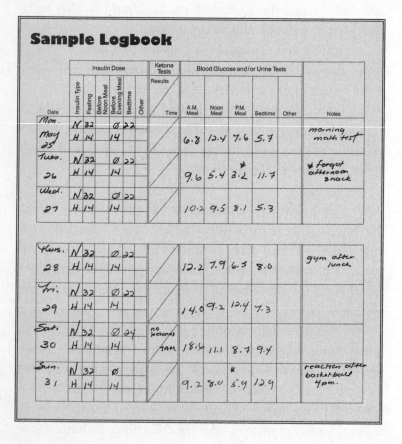

Sample Logbook

Date	Insulin Dose						Ketone Tests	Blood Glucose and/or Urine Tests					Notes
	Insulin Type	Fasting	Before Noon Meal	Before Evening Meal	Bedtime	Other	Results / Time	A.M. Meal	Noon Meal	P.M. Meal	Bedtime	Other	
Mon. May 25	N 32 H 14		Ø 14	22				6.8	12.4	7.6	5.7		morning math test
Tues. 26	N 32 H 14		Ø 14	22				9.6	5.4	3.2 *	11.7		* forgot afternoon snack
Wed. 27	N 32 H 14		Ø 14	22				10.2	9.5	8.1	5.3		
Thurs. 28	N 32 H 14		Ø 14	22				12.2	7.9	6.5	8.0		gym after lunch
Fri. 29	N 32 H 14		Ø 14	22				14.0	9.2	12.4	7.3		
Sat. 30	N 32 H 14		Ø 14	24			no ketones 7AM	18.6	11.1	8.7	9.4		
Sun. 31	N 32 H 14		Ø 14					9.2	8.0	5.9 *	12.9		reaction after basketball 4pm.

The Three-Month Test

The hemoglobin A1C test is a measure of the average blood glucose level over the previous three months. This test is also known as glycosylated or glycated hemoglobin or glycohe-moglobin. In our discussion we simply refer to hemoglobin A1C checking as A1C.

Hemoglobin is the part of the red blood cell that carries oxygen from the lungs to the rest of the body. Scientists have discovered that in all people, whether they have diabetes or not, some glucose sticks to the hemoglobin and stays there for the lifespan of the red blood cell—about three to four months. The amount of glucose that sticks to the hemoglobin reflects the average blood glucose level during that period, and can be measured in a laboratory using the A1C test. When the average blood glucose level has been high, the test result will be high. Thus, the A1C indicates the level of control over the previous few months. The level of A1C achieved over time is the best predictor we have of the risk of long-term diabetes-related complications, such as eye, kidney, or nerve damage.

What A1C Levels Mean in Terms of Average Blood Glucose Concentrations

A1C	mmol/L	mg/dL
5%	5.0	90
6%	6.5–7.0	115–125
7%	8.0–9.0	145–160
8%	9.5–11.0	170–200
9%	11.0–13.0	200–240
10%	12.5–15.0	230–270
11%	14.0–17.0	250–300
12%	15.5–19.0	280–350

A1C can be measured at any time, and often enough blood can be collected for this test from a finger prick, although sometimes the blood sample has to be taken from a vein. There are different methods for measuring A1C. Some methods give immediate results; others take a little longer. Efforts are now underway to standardize A1C worldwide. In people without diabetes A1C levels are generally in the range of about 4 to 6 percent. Nonetheless you'll want to check the non-diabetic range for your laboratory. Even with intensive treatment, few children and teens with diabetes can achieve this level without risking frequent low blood glucose reactions. Instead, strive to achieve the best A1C levels possible. In the absence of many low blood glucose reactions, levels less than or equal to 7 percent are considered to be target range for adolescents (13 years and older) and adults with diabetes and reflect excellent control; for children aged 6 to 12 years, A1C levels less than 8 percent are in target, and for children 5 years and under, levels less than 8.5 percent are considered to be in target range. Generally speaking, A1C levels between 8 and 10 percent suggest a need for problem solving with the team and extra effort to improve control, and levels more than 10 percent are a worry and indicate a need for concerted effort by child, family, and team to avoid trouble.

Children should have their A1C measured every three months and the results should be recorded to chart overall progress. Be sure to note when a different lab than the usual

Table 5.1 Age-Specific Targets for Blood Glucose Levels and A1C Levels According to Canadian Diabetes Association Clinical Practice Guidelines 2008

Age	Target Pre-Meal Blood Glucose Level	Target A1C Level
5 years and under	6–12 mmol/L (110–220 mg/dL)	less than 8.5%
6–12 years	4–10 mmol/L (70–180 mg/dL)	less than 8.0%
Over 12 years	4–8 mmol/L (70–145 mg/dL)	less than 7.0%

one processes the test—methods, and therefore results, can differ from lab to lab, giving an inaccurate picture of progress.

Children and teens using insulin pump therapy may be able to aim for lower blood glucose targets and achieve lower A1C levels. Speak with your diabetes team about the best possible targets for your child.

Adjusting Insulin Doses

As children grow and their appetites and activity levels change, their need for insulin also changes. You shouldn't have to wait for a regular appointment with someone on the diabetes team to respond to these changes. Who better to monitor the changing patterns in the child's blood glucose level and overall health than the family? Studies show that parents and children who actively participate in the diabetes management process are the most successful in adapting to the disease.

Remember that the need for more insulin or more injections does not mean a child's diabetes is getting worse. Similarly, a decrease in insulin doesn't mean the diabetes is going away. Adjusting insulin to the body's current demands is simply a way of maintaining good balance and achieving better control. For example, a heavier child may need more insulin than a smaller child, and a child who is always on the go may need less insulin than a child who is not as active. A teenager will likely require more insulin during puberty than after the growth spurt. People generally need more insulin when they are sick than when they are well and students may require more insulin during exam week, because of the increased stress.

To make independent insulin dose adjustments, be they temporary or permanent, parents and teens must:
- be confident that blood glucose checks are accurate and meal plans are being followed (i.e., no secret snacking or skipping meals)

- know the child's blood glucose target range
- understand the actions of the insulin being used
- understand what each blood glucose check means
- know when to contact the health care team

How to Think and Talk about Insulin Dose Adjustment

You will have lots of time to learn about and practice insulin dose adjustment together with your diabetes educator as your coach. In the section that follows we'll give you some ways of talking about insulin and insulin dose changes. Having a common understanding of what we mean by terms such as basic dose, basal, and bolus will help with our discussion about insulin dose adjustment.

The Basic Insulin Dose: This is the type and amount of insulin dose that your child receives when her blood glucose is in target. For example Chantal's *basic insulin dose* at breakfast time is NPH 15 units and Humalog 3 units.

Correction: A temporary change in the rapid-acting insulin. Chantal's blood glucose levels are normally in target at breakfast time so she takes her basic dose of NPH 15 and Humalog 3 units most days. But let us say that today she wakes up with a blood glucose level of 13 mmol/L (230 mg/dL), which is 3 mmol/L (55 mg/dL) above the upper limit of her target range. Chantal's parents have learned to correct "out of target" blood glucose levels by giving Chantal an extra unit of rapid-acting Humalog for every 3 mmol/L (55 mg/dL) above target. This formula is called a *correction* factor. Today she needs to take her basic insulin dose of NPH 15 units and Humalog 4 units (3 units for her basic insulin dose plus 1 unit to correct the high blood glucose level). Similarly, Chantal's parents make a temporary reduction in the Humalog when the blood glucose level is too low. Chantal's family uses a correction factor for these temporary adjustments. Other families learn to use a variable insulin dose scale (sometimes called a "scale" or "insulin algorithm") to make the corrections. The purpose is the same; that is, a consistent approach to corrections in order to bring the blood glucose level back into target by the next mealtime.

What Does a 10 Percent Dose Adjustment Mean?

If the child is on:	adjust by:
less than 20 units of insulin/day	1 unit at a time
20–30 units/day	2 units at a time
30–40 units/day	3 units at a time
over 40 units/day	4 units at a time

Insulin Dose Adjustment: A change in the dose of insulin based on a pattern of blood glucose levels taken during a number of days. The rapid- and/or the intermediate- or long-acting insulin may be adjusted as needed. Such adjustments are common in children especially at the beginning and end of the honeymoon, as the child grows or finishes growing, and when a change of season leads to altered levels of activity, e.g., the arrival of spring with longer daylight hours. For example, Chantal's blood glucose level before breakfast has been higher than 10 mmol/L (180 mg/dL) for three days in a row. Each morning her parents have given her extra rapid-acting insulin to get her blood glucose back down by lunch hour. Now it is time to do an overall adjustment in her insulin dose so she no longer wakes up with a high blood glucose result. Her parents have learned to increase her bedtime NPH to reduce her blood glucose levels through the night so that Chantal has a better chance of waking up with blood glucose levels that are in target.

Temporary Dose Adjustment: A temporary change in insulin dose to compensate for a temporary change in food or activity, or to deal with an illness. The rapid-acting and/or intermediate-acting or long-acting insulin may be changed. It is assumed that the circumstances creating the need for the insulin dose adjustment are out of the ordinary and will go away and the insulin requirements will return to the "basic dose."

When to Make Adjustments
People with diabetes know when change is required by the way they feel, and by the results of their blood glucose and urine ketone checks. Provided they are sticking to the meal plan reasonably well and/or using their insulin to carbohydrate ratio accurately, continuous high blood glucose readings usually mean that more insulin is required; repeated low readings usually mean that less insulin is needed. Generally speaking, you can assume that the insulin dose is right and no permanent change in the basic dose is necessary when:
• the child feels well and is free of symptoms of high or low blood glucose
• the urine is free of ketones
• 70 to 80 percent of the blood glucose checks are within the target range

With any insulin regimen, be it two, three, or four or more injections a day, it is important to know which insulin is acting when, and therefore which insulin dose needs to be changed when glucose levels are either too high or too low.

Jane is a 10-year-old who has had diabetes for five years. She receives NPH and Humalog insulin before breakfast, Humalog at supper, and NPH at bedtime. Jane's family has learned that each of the four daily blood checks is dependent on the action of one of the four insulin doses:

- the breakfast reading tells them how well the bedtime NPH from the night before is working
- the lunch reading indicates the effectiveness of the breakfast Humalog insulin
- the supper reading reflects the action of the breakfast NPH
- the bedtime reading tells them if the supper Humalog insulin is working

These guidelines may seem a little simplistic, but they're a good starting point for Jane and her family when her blood checks are off target. When Jane woke up with high readings three mornings in a row, her parents knew she needed more NPH (intermediate-acting) insulin at night. When she had a couple of nights when she was low before her bedtime snack, her parents decreased her Humalog (rapid-acting) dose at suppertime.

Carol is a 16-year-old grade 10 student and a competitive swimmer. She's had diabetes for eight months and has been on long-acting Levemir at bedtime and rapid-acting NovoRapid before each meal and snack from the beginning. This routine allows her to have the flexibility she needs for her busy schedule without compromising her control. She checks her blood glucose at least four or five times a day. Each check gives her specific information about the effectiveness of a particular dose of insulin. Specifically,

- the pre-breakfast blood glucose result reflects the effectiveness of the long-acting Levemir
- the lunchtime reading reflects the effectiveness of the breakfast time NovoRapid
- the afternoon snack reading tells her how well the lunchtime NovoRapid worked
- the suppertime check reflects the effectiveness of the afternoon snack time insulin

- the bedtime check gives good information about how well the suppertime insulin worked

Adjusting the Basic Insulin Dose Based on Pattern Management

Most people aim to keep blood glucose levels in the target range 70 to 80 percent of the time. Some variability is to be expected. The basic insulin dose should be changed only when a pattern or trend of blood glucose results are outside of the target range. If the child is feeling well and has no ketones, it is time to make an insulin dose adjustment when the blood glucose is high at the same time of day for three days in a row, or low at the same time of day for two days in a row or three times in a week. If there is good reason for the highs and lows—such as unexpected extra exercise that wasn't allowed for—the dose adjustment may be delayed a while longer, to see if the pattern persists.

Specific Guidelines for Insulin Dose Adjustment

In Tables 5.2 and 5.3 you will find guidelines for when and how to adjust the basic dose of insulin for those patients taking two or three injections of rapid- and intermediate-acting insulin. They go along with the diabetes education program at The Hospital for Sick Children, Toronto. If you are not part of the Hospital for Sick Children Program, please discuss these guidelines with your doctor or diabetes nurse before using them.

These guidelines should be used only if the child feels well and there are no ketones in the blood or urine—in which case more immediate action is required. Ketones should be checked when the blood glucose is more than 13 mmol or 230 mg/dL.

Once you have decided to change the basic insulin dose, adjustments of 10 percent of the specific dose are generally suggested. For example, a morning dose of 20 NPH may be increased to 22. Once you have changed the dose you need wait only two days to see if it works before changing it again. Once you arrive at a dose that gets the appropriate blood glucose into target that becomes your new basic dose.

Table 5.2 Adjusting the Insulin Dose for Those on Intermediate- and Rapid-Acting Insulin Twice a Day—before Breakfast and Supper

Time of Day	Blood Glucose	Time Frame	Action	Insulin Dose
Before Breakfast	Above Target	3 days in a row	Increase	Supper Intermediate
Before Lunch	Above Target	3 days in a row	Increase	Morning Rapid
Before Supper	Above Target	3 days in a row	Increase	Morning Intermediate
Before Bedtime Snack	Above Target	3 days in a row	Increase	Supper Rapid
Before Breakfast	Below Target	2 days in a row	Decrease	Supper Intermediate
Before Lunch	Below Target	2 days in a row	Decrease	Morning Rapid
Before Supper	Below Target	2 days in a row	Decrease	Morning Intermediate
Before Bedtime Snack	Below Target	2 days in a row	Decrease	Supper Rapid

Note: This routine is most common in infants and toddlers. Over time these children will be able to achieve better blood glucose control with more frequent injections.

Traditionally, diabetes management for children and teens has consisted of taking insulin two or three times a day, monitoring blood glucose three to four times a day, following a meal plan that involves eating the same amount of food at around the same time each day, and compensating for extra activity with extra food.

Today, a more proactive approach is increasingly used by people of all ages who have diabetes. People are encourage to learn to "think like a pancreas"; to try not only to correct blood glucose levels that go out of target but also to try to match their injected or infused insulin to the food that they eat and activity that they do, so that blood glucoses remain in target as much as possible. This approach that we used to call

Table 5.3 Three Times Daily Injection: Intermediate at Breakfast and Bedtime and Rapid-Acting Insulin at Breakfast and Suppertime

Time of Day	Blood glucose	Time Frame	Action	Insulin Dose
Before Breakfast	Above Target	3 days in a row	Increase	Bedtime Intermediate
Before Lunch	Above Target	3 days in a row	Increase	Morning Rapid
Before Supper	Above Target	3 days in a row	Increase	Morning Intermediate
Before Bedtime Snack	Above Target	3 days in a row	Increase	Supper Rapid
Before Breakfast	Below Target	2 days in a row	Decrease	Bedtime Intermediate
Before Lunch	Below Target	2 days in a row	Decrease	Morning Rapid
Before Supper	Below Target	2 days in a row	Decrease	Morning Intermediate
Before Bedtime Snack	Below Target	2 days in a row	Decrease	Supper Rapid

"intensive management" is now considered to be conventional or usual treatment.

The extra work required pays off in that it allows a more flexible schedule without compromising safety or control. It's like flying a jumbo jet compared to a one-engine plane—it may be more complex but there is also more potential. People can vary their activities more, and don't have to eat meals at the same time every day because they are taking insulin before every meal. Through either four or more daily injections, or an insulin infusion pump, this approach aims to provide a steady stream of insulin day and night—more the way a pancreas does—and extra insulin with food.

Here's how it works. Rapid-acting insulin is taken with each meal, breakfast, lunch, and dinner, and often with an afternoon or evening snack. Intermediate- or long-acting insulin is usually taken at bedtime. Some people choose to take the long-acting insulin at another time of the day, e.g., suppertime—for safety reasons, however, this is not advised with intermediate-acting insulin. The dose of the rapid-acting insulin is based on the current blood glucose level, the amount of carbohydrate about to be consumed, and the activity planned during the next 2 to 3 hours. Thus, when the pre-meal blood glucose goes higher than the upper limit of target, which is usually 7 mmol/L (125 mg/dL) for most older children and teens, there is an opportunity to give some additional rapid-acting insulin right then, to bring the blood glucose back into the target range. Likewise, if the blood glucose level is less than 4 mmol/L (70 mg/dL) just prior to a meal, or if a lot of exercise is planned in the next few hours, the insulin dose can be reduced immediately.

This more intensive approach to diabetes management was central to the groundbreaking Diabetes Control and

Complications Trial (DCCT)—a multicenter study (funded by the U.S. government) that looked at the effects of tight blood glucose control on the risk of diabetes complications. In this study, more than 1,400 volunteers, 13–39 years of age, were divided into two groups. One group managed their diabetes with what was then called intensified therapy, while the other group continued with traditional therapy, one to three injections per day. At the end of the study's nine-year period, the two groups were compared. The intensified therapy group showed an average A1C reading of 7.2 percent, which is significantly lower than the traditional treatment group's average of 8.9 percent. The intensified therapy group had fewer signs of complications from diabetes: diabetic eye disease (retinopathy) had started in only one-quarter as many people as in the control group; kidney disease (nephropathy) occurred in only half as many; nerve disease (neuropathy) in only one-third as many. Of those who received intensified management and who had shown early signs of these three complications before the study began, far fewer showed progression of the complications.

The good news is that good control pays off in terms of short- and long-term health. Attempting to do whatever is possible to get a good match between insulin and food and activity usually results in the best possible control for a specific child at a particular time of his life and stage of development. Not all children or families will be ready for four or more injections a day or an insulin pump from the beginning. All the same, it is important to value excellent control and optimize the routine that your child is on so that the best possible control is achieved. Four or more insulin injections may be ideal but remember that even if your child is only on rapid-acting insulin twice a day, you still have two opportunities to correct a high or low blood glucose level and you can still look for patterns to adjust the overall insulin dose. As new tools and insulins are developed, and as your child matures, try to keep an open mind to changes that your team may recommend.

In Table 5.4 you will find guidelines for when and how to adjust the basic dose of insulin for those patients on a multiple daily insulin regimen.

Insulin Dose Adjustment for Children and Teens on Insulin Pumps

When diabetes is managed with the insulin pump, children and teens and their parents need to learn how to adjust both basal insulin rate(s) and bolus doses. You may recall that the insulin pump delivers a tiny trickle of insulin constantly, day and night, and that this is called the basal insulin rate. It is common for people with diabetes to require more basal insulin at certain times of the day and to have more than one basal insulin rate programmed into the pump. You may also remember that people who manage their diabetes with a pump give themselves extra insulin with meals or to correct a high blood glucose by selecting a dose and pushing a button on the pump to release that dose through the tiny cannula and into the body. This extra insulin is called the bolus dose, which is calculated to match the food intake and to correct blood glucose levels outside of the target range. As previously explained, the formula used to calculate how much insulin to take for a given amount of food is called the *insulin to carbohydrate ratio*. In other words, how many grams of carbohydrate will 1 unit of insulin cover? The insulin to carbohydrate ratio will vary from one person to the next and may even vary in the same person from one time of the day to another. For example, Marcus uses an insulin to carbohydrate ratio of 1 unit of insulin for 8 grams of carbohydrate at breakfast and 1 unit for 10 grams of carbohydrate at other times of the day.

Table 5.4 Intermediate- or Long-Acting Insulin at Bedtime; Rapid-Acting Insulin with Meals and Snacks (Three or More Injections Per Day)

Time of Day	Blood glucose	Time Frame	Action	Insulin Dose
Before Breakfast	Above Target	3 days in a row	Increase	Bedtime Intermediate or Long-Acting
Before Lunch	Above Target	3 days in a row	Increase	Breakfast Rapid-Acting
Before Afternoon Snack or Early Supper	Above Target	3 days in a row	Increase	Lunchtime Rapid-Acting
Before Late Supper	Above Target	3 days in a row	Increase	Snack Time Rapid-Acting
Before Bedtime Snack	Above Target	3 days in a row	Increase	Supper Rapid-Acting
Before Breakfast	Below Target	2 days in a row	Decrease	Bedtime Intermediate-Acting
Before Lunch	Below Target	2 days in a row	Decrease	Morning Rapid-Acting
Before Afternoon Snack or Early Supper	Below Target	2 days in a row	Decrease	Morning Intermediate-Acting
Before Late Dinner	Below Target	2 days in a row	Decrease	Snack Time Insulin if insulin is taken with snack
Before Bedtime Snack	Below Target	2 days in a row	Decrease	Supper Rapid-Acting

Note: It is possible for the long-acting insulin to be given at a regular time of the day, other than bedtime. All the same, the best blood glucose check to evaluate the effectiveness of the long-acting insulin is the pre-breakfast result. Blood glucose checks during the day when there has been a span of time longer than 4 hours without carbohydrate or rapid-acting insulin are also useful in assessing the effectiveness of the long-acting insulin.

In addition to taking bolus insulin with food, people on pumps learn to take extra insulin when their blood glucose level is high and to reduce insulin when blood glucose is low. This means figuring out how much insulin is required to bring the blood glucose back into the target range during the next few hours. For example, Marcus's blood glucose before lunch is 12 mmol/L (220 mg/dL). At a previous clinic visit his doctor helped Marcus figure out that it takes 1 unit of insulin to reduce his blood glucose by 3 mmol/L (55 mg/dL). This is called the *correction factor*. Marcus's correction factor is 3. This means that if he wants his pre-lunch blood glucose of 12 mmol/L (220 mg/dL) to get to his target of 6 mmol/L (110 mg/dL) he needs to bolus 2 units of rapid-acting insulin in addition to the insulin required for his meal. Most teens and parents learn how to program the basic basal and bolus insulin information into the pump. By checking blood glucose results before meals and 2 hours after meals and recording the results, it is possible (and important) for those on pumps to be on the lookout for patterns and to make overall changes in the basic insulin doses. When parents or teens discover a period of three days in a row where the levels are high at the same time of the day, or two days when they are low at the same time of the day, an insulin adjustment should be considered. As with other insulin regimens, once teens or parents determine that an adjustment is required they learn to change the dose every second day until one of the readings comes into target. This dose becomes the new basic dose. Target blood glucose for most people on pumps are between 4–7 mmol/L (70–125 mg/dL) before meals and 5–8 mmol/L (90–145 mg/dL) 2 hours after meals.

In summary

- The blood glucose result before breakfast indicates the effectiveness of the night-time basal.
- Blood glucose results done 2 hours after meals indicate the effectiveness of the mealtime bolus.

- Blood glucose checks done 4 or more hours after meals and/or correction bolus doses are good indicators of the effectiveness of basal rates in the few hours before the blood glucose check.
- Blood glucose results done 2 hours after correcting a high blood glucose indicate the effectiveness of the correction factor.

Adjusting Insulin and Food for Planned Activity

Most children welcome routines, but once in a while schedules change, and without adequate planning the blood glucose balance may be upset. A weekly swimming lesson on Sunday morning, for example, will create different insulin demands than a weekly piano lesson on Monday afternoon. Parents, and in time children, can learn to assess the impact of these regular events, and when an opportunity for a new activity comes along, everyone will be better able to cope with the change.

Because exercise both lowers blood glucose and increases the speed of insulin absorption, it's a good idea to match it, whenever possible, with extra food. After a while, you'll become more familiar with how the child responds to activity and you'll have a better idea of how much food, if any, to offer. Some (usually older) children learn to decrease insulin on days of extra activity rather than taking extra food.

- In general, provide extra food for extra exercise. Children need about 10 to 15 grams of carbohydrate (such as a 4-ounce [125 mL] juice box, or half a sandwich) for every 30 minutes of activity outside the usual. If possible, monitor blood glucose levels before and after the activity—these levels will provide important information for future activities. For example, if the glucose level is very high after an activity, then less (or no) extra food may be needed. If the glucose level is low, even more snacks will be required.

- Always make sure children have enough rapid-acting glucose with them (such as glucose tablets, fruit roll-ups, juice boxes, or granola bars), especially if the activity goes on a long time or is off the beaten track.
- If the child starts to experience a low blood glucose reaction, stop the activity immediately and treat the reaction. Don't resume the activity until the symptoms have resolved and the child has eaten some extra food.

Preventing Delayed Low Blood Glucose

- Monitor blood glucose levels long after exercise. Lows can occur up to 12 hours later.
- Children doing activities after supper should have a bigger evening snack. Doing a midnight or middle-of-the-night (2 to 4 a.m.) check will help detect late-night lows.

Twelve-year-old Michele has always taken her ballet lesson on Saturday afternoon. To get ready for an exam, she's planning to add an extra hour to the lesson. In preparation for the change in her schedule, Michele's parents consider her current routine. Michele always has an afternoon snack of a fruit and starch. The extended class means that she'll be dancing at the time when her morning intermediate-acting (NPH) insulin is reaching its peak. Michele will be home for her usual 6:00 p.m. supper. Without the extra class, her blood glucose level is usually between 8 and 12 mmol/L (145–220 mg/dL) at suppertime. However, her blood glucose level often drops in the night after vigorous exercise late in the day. Michele's parents work out the following plan:

- Eat an extra fruit and starch choice prior to her second hour of dance.
- Take blood glucose monitoring equipment to the lesson, as

well as a small juice box and granola bar, in case her blood glucose starts to drop during the lesson.

- Check the blood glucose level at the end of the class to evaluate the effectiveness of the plan.
- Eat an additional starch choice at bedtime to offset the delayed effects of the exercise.

Another choice would be to decrease the morning dose of NPH by about 20 percent. Frequent monitoring will be necessary to determine the effect of this adjustment, and to detect or prevent hypoglycemia.

Q&A

My 15-year-old daughter's pre-dinner blood glucose checks are either high or missing most of the time. I suspect that she's snacking on the way home from school and that's why her blood glucose is a little high. Any ideas about how to approach this?
You're wise not to demand explanations for why every test result is the way it is—or to accuse your daughter of cheating. This is a sure way to get no blood glucose readings, or made up results. On the other hand, it is risky to increase the insulin dose if you're not confident that the readings are accurate. It could be that the checks are done just a short while after your daughter has been snacking. Some parents deal with this situation by saying to their teen, "It seems your blood glucose checks are high before supper. Let's put our heads together to figure out what kinds of adjustments might be necessary." This gives you an opportunity to explore some of the factors that may be contributing to the high level, such as being hungry and eating more right after school or on the way home. Then the right kind of adjustments can be made.

Should I let my son continue to play in day-long soccer tournaments? What about the walkathon next month?
One of the most important steps in helping children cope with diabetes is minimizing change in their lifestyle. Your son should continue to participate in all the activities he enjoys. Even if all-day soccer tournaments are new to his list of activities, there's still no need to ban them. If you cut out soccer tournaments, something your son presumably enjoys, you'll increase any resentment he may have toward the disease, and perhaps toward you. You can prepare him for a day-long tournament, or next month's walkathon, by providing lots of snacks and monitoring his blood glucose in as subtle a way as possible. To start, at least, you should also give a little less insulin on these days. Once you see the effect of the extra activity on his glucose levels, you can decide whether less insulin, more food, or a combination of both is the best way to go. Consult your diabetes team for more advice.

Is it all right to scuba dive?
Scuba diving may be dangerous for people with diabetes, because of the risk of becoming hypoglycemic underwater and not being able to respond by taking glucose, causing a mild insulin reaction to escalate into a severe one. However, hard and fast restrictions don't work. At present, divers with diabetes are advised to consult a doctor experienced in dive medicine, to learn everything they can about taking the necessary safety precautions. Make sure that you recognize the risks involved, and that your dive buddy knows the risks, too. For the latest information on the subject, call the Divers Alert Network (DAN) at Duke University Medical Center, 1-800-446-2671. Or check their website at www.diversalertnetwork.org.

When my son's blood glucose is high, I send him outside to run around the block. He seems to resent the fact that his sister gets to continue her regular activities while his are disrupted. Is there any way to get around this problem?

While exercise does tend to counteract high blood glucose levels, exercise and activity should not be considered a tool of diabetes treatment. There are other ways that might work just as well. Try sitting down with your son and coming up with alternatives. For instance, if this is happening at the same time every day, maybe you need to increase the insulin dose that would affect this glucose reading.

My teenage daughter thinks she's too heavy. She's been exercising 4 to 6 hours a day trying to lose weight. Is this healthy for her?

No. Most people do not lose weight when they increase their activity level—they seem to take in an increased amount of food to offset the fuel burned by the exercise. Excessive amounts of exercise in a teenage girl wanting to lose weight may be one of the first signs that she is unduly worried about her body image and possibly developing an eating disorder. Discuss your concern with your family doctor and members of your diabetes team.

Our family is very athletic, and I expect our 6-year-old son has a lot of potential, too. How can we encourage him to explore athletics without being intimidated by his diabetes?

Introduce your son to sports slowly, and increase his exposure as he shows more interest. Many professional and skilled amateur athletes have diabetes. Your local support group may be able to provide a list. Encourage your son to write to athletes with diabetes and to use them as role models. Many athletes find the time to write a note back, which can be all the encouragement a child needs.

SIX

Handling the Highs and the Lows, Including Sick Days

Jacob knew he should stop and take a break from the squash game, but he was having too much fun. And besides, he was winning for a change. "Are you sure you don't want to stop and have some juice?" his brother Paul asked. "You've been working pretty hard."

"You're just trying to avoid losing," Jacob kidded. A few minutes passed and Paul insisted they stop for a juice break.

"Look, I know when I need a break," said Jacob sharply, no longer kidding. "Let's just keep playing." Suddenly he was feeling a little light-headed and weak in the knees. Paul noticed that Jacob was getting paler and paler and ran to get some orange juice from his sports bag. Within a few minutes of drinking the juice Jacob's color began to return to normal.

Jacob has a low blood glucose reaction at least once or twice a week. Most of the time he recognizes them and treats them without incident. But sometimes, when he gets caught up in friendly competition, he pushes himself beyond safe limits. Luckily, his brother knew the signs—first angry and defensive, then clammy and faint. If he hadn't gotten treatment at that point, Jacob might have become confused, drowsy, and unable to take anything by mouth.

It's been said that managing diabetes is a little like performing a complicated juggling act. Sometimes the ball drops. No matter how hard you try, it's impossible to keep the blood glucose in target range all of the time. Sometimes it will be high, other times low. Often there is no explanation for the results. This chapter covers the extremes:

- hypoglycemia, or low blood glucose, often referred to as an insulin reaction or insulin shock
- hyperglycemia, or high blood glucose
- diabetic ketoacidosis (DKA), the result of a severe shortage of insulin
- sick days, leading to either hypoglycemia or DKA when not handled properly

Hypoglycemia (Low Blood Glucose or Insulin Reaction)

A blood glucose level lower than about 3.3 mmol/L (60 mg/dL) is defined as hypoglycemia. The feelings associated with hypoglycemia are called an "insulin reaction."

The earliest symptoms of low blood glucose may resemble the feelings many people experience when they've gone without food for a long time: they may feel hungry, tired, and irritable, and they may even have a headache. These early warning signs tell us that the body needs glucose quickly. As the blood glucose continues to drop, other signs and symptoms may develop—shakiness, pale skin, cold sweat, dilated pupils, and pounding heart. These result from the body's attempt to boost the blood glucose from within. Certain hormones, including glucagon, adrenaline, cortisol, and others, urge our liver and muscles to convert stored glucose into glucose, which enters the bloodstream.

In someone without diabetes, the body turns off the insulin supply whenever blood glucose is at a normal level, or below normal. But in people with diabetes, the injected insulin continues to work; as fast as the glucose enters the bloodstream, the insulin pushes it into the cells, so the level of glucose in the blood remains low until the person takes glucose by mouth.

Most people with type 1 diabetes experience low blood glucose reactions from time to time. Indeed, mild reactions that are easily recognized and treated, without too much interruption in activities, should be expected. They can be seen as the price paid for good blood glucose control. Note that some people experience symptoms of hypoglycemia even when their blood glucose level is higher than 4 mmol/L (72 mg/dL).

Common Signs and Symptoms of a Mild Insulin Reaction

- shakiness—"butterflies," feeling nervous for no reason
- cold, clammy sweatiness, unlike sweat from playing hard
- dilated pupils, "funny-looking" eyes
- mood change—irritable, grouchy, impatient; temper tantrums in younger children
- hunger, and sometimes nausea due to the hunger
- lack of energy—tired, weak, floppy
- lack of concentration
- blurred vision
- pounding heart
- change in skin color—pale, most noticeably in the face and around the mouth

- poor sleep patterns—restlessness, crying out, sleepwalking, or nightmares

Usually insulin reactions happen suddenly, over a period of minutes rather than hours. While they may occur at any time of the day or night, they happen most often when insulin is working at its peak.

Although low blood glucose symptoms vary from child to child, each child tends to develop his or her own set of symptoms. After one or two episodes, parents and children learn to recognize an insulin reaction quickly. It is helpful for parents and older children to explain the child's specific symptoms to teachers, coaches, school bus drivers, and other caregivers. Even young children can be taught to alert an adult to these symptoms, by using a specific phrase such as "I feel funny" or "I need glucose."

Hypoglycemia may be most difficult to detect in infants or toddlers, who are unable to describe their feelings. A sudden change in behavior, with irritability, crying, pale face, and "floppiness," may be the tip-off that blood glucose is too low.

Treatment of Mild Insulin Reaction

Insulin reactions, even mild ones, must be treated right away. Always have a source of fast-acting sugar available, such as juice, dextrose tablets, or even table glucose. In the event of an insulin reaction, follow these steps:

- If possible, check the blood glucose level to confirm hypoglycemia. A blood glucose level lower than 6 mmol/L (110 mg/dL), accompanied by symptoms of low blood glucose, should be treated. (If you are unable to check the blood glucose before treating the reaction, check it as soon as possible afterward. Note the response to treatment.)
- Give a source of fast-acting glucose; about 10 to 15 grams of

carbohydrate is all it takes to treat an insulin reaction. Examples include: 4 ounces (125 mL) of unsweetened juice or regular soft drink, or two to three dextrose tablets, or 8 ounces (250 mL) of milk, or 2 teaspoons (10 mL) of sugar. Babies and toddlers require about half this amount and it is best offered in the form of juice or milk. Various forms of prepackaged glucose may be available from your pharmacy or diabetes supply shop. Read the label ahead of time to determine the amount you should give to treat a low blood glucose reaction. We generally recommend an amount that will supply 10 to 15 grams of carbohydrate. If a mild reaction occurs just before a meal or snack, start the meal or snack immediately, beginning with some simple carbohydrate.

- Wait for the sugar to take effect. This is the hardest part. People who experience hypoglycemia feel extremely hungry and scared. They are often tempted to continue to eat and drink until the symptoms go away. This may result in a high blood glucose level later in the day. If symptoms persist, recheck the blood glucose in 10 to 15 minutes. If it is still low, the child should have an extra 10 to 15 grams of carbohydrate. If vigorous exercise is anticipated prior to the next meal or snack, or if the reaction occurs during the night, the simple carbohydrate should be followed with a complex carbohydrate (one from the starch group).
- Attempt to determine the cause of the insulin reaction. If there is no apparent reason, consider reducing the appropriate insulin by 10 to 20 percent the next day.
- Note the blood glucose levels, time, response, and possible cause of the reaction in your logbook.

Note: IF IN DOUBT, TREAT. When you can't check the blood glucose level to confirm an insulin reaction, give glucose anyway just to be safe.

Why Do Insulin Reactions Occur?

Understanding the reasons for hypoglycemia is key to preventing it. Causes are usually related to the three major factors affecting blood glucose balance: insulin, food, and activity.

Too Much Insulin

How can it happen that children get too much insulin? Well, mistakes do happen. Sometimes children get the wrong type of insulin or take the wrong amount at the wrong time. Other times parents forget to reduce the insulin when the blood glucose levels are consistently under the target level at a particular time of the day.

Not Enough Food

This can happen easily enough—for example, when children get caught up in their activities and forget to eat, when toddlers sleep through snack time or when teens sleep through breakfast or skip a meal.

Too Much Unplanned Activity

This is the most frequent cause of hypoglycemia, because children aren't accustomed to planning ahead before they jump into an active game like tag or soccer. That's why the blood glucose target range is wider in younger children than in adults; it allows for such spontaneity. Children should be able to enjoy any sport or activity with planning.

Severe Hypoglycemic Reaction

Occasionally a severe hypoglycemic reaction occurs when early symptoms of low blood glucose go undetected and untreated. Know what to look for and what to do in case a severe low blood glucose reaction develops.

Signs and Symptoms of a Severe Insulin Reaction
- "drunken-like behavior"—slurred speech, staggering, confusion, combativeness
- low energy—extremely tired, difficult to wake up
- loss of consciousness
- convulsions or seizures
- temporary paralysis down one side of the body

Treatment of a Severe Insulin Reaction
This is an emergency situation. Anyone showing signs of a severe insulin reaction needs immediate help. The blood glucose is dangerously low, therefore the child needs sugar. However, someone who is very drowsy, unconscious, or having a convulsion or seizure must not be given juice or any other liquid by mouth, because of the risk of choking. Rather, the child should be turned onto her side to prevent choking, and glucagon (see below) should be injected. If a glucagon emergency kit is not available, an ambulance should be called and the child transported to the closest hospital emergency department, where either a glucose-containing solution will be injected intravenously, or glucagon will be given. While you wait for the ambulance, honey or corn syrup may be rubbed on the lips, gums, or lining of the child's mouth.

About Glucagon
You will be taught how to inject glucagon should your child ever have low blood sugar and not be able to swallow because of drowsiness or unconsciousness. Glucagon is a hormone that stimulates the liver to release glucose into the bloodstream. It must be injected. When glucagon acts on the liver, the blood glucose level rises and the child begins to rouse within about 15 minutes. Families of all children with type 1 diabetes should

have usable (not expired) glucagon on hand, and know where it's kept and how to use it. A glucagon emergency kit consists of a small vial containing dry glucagon powder and a pre-filled glass syringe containing sterile diluting solution. The contents of the syringe and vial should be mixed only when they are about to be used. Keep the kit in an agreed-upon place so everyone can find it easily.

An injection of glucagon can only help. It can never be harmful. It is impossible to overdose on glucagon. Parents who think their child may need glucagon should play it safe and give the injection.

Preparing and Giving Glucagon

- Remove the flip-off seal from the vial (bottle) of glucagon.
- Remove the needle protector from the syringe and inject the entire contents of the syringe into the vial of glucagon.
- Shake vial gently until glucagon dissolves and the solution becomes clear. There is no need to remove the needle from the vial while shaking the bottle.
- Using the same syringe, withdraw all of the solution from the vial.
- For children 6 years of age and older, inject all of the solution (1 mL), just as you would inject insulin. Children under 6 may require only half the mixed dose (0.5 mL), as recommended by the doctor or diabetes nurse. Some clinics may recommend an even smaller dose. Mini doses of glucagon, discussed in the section on sick day management, should not be used to treat a severe hypoglycemic reaction.

After the glucagon has been injected, check the blood glucose and observe the child carefully. Make sure the child is turned on her side to avoid choking. Usually it takes about 5 to 20 minutes for the child to wake up. If not, the child should be taken to the closest hospital emergency department. Once the child is fully awake, offer some juice or a glucose-containing soft drink. Recheck the blood glucose and notify the doctor. We know that one severe reaction makes the person with diabetes more susceptible to another reaction in the next 24–48 hours. Therefore the appropriate insulin dose should be reduced about 20 percent for at least the next day or two to prevent another episode.

Either the severe hypoglycemic reaction or the use of glucagon can trigger nausea or vomiting, especially in children. They may be unable to eat or drink afterward. If this occurs:

- Recheck blood glucose levels immediately.
- If you are able to reach the doctor, she can advise you on whether to proceed to the hospital.
- If you cannot reach the doctor, go to the nearest hospital, even if the blood glucose levels are starting to rise.

Remember, a glucagon kit doesn't do any good if no one knows where it's kept or how to use it.

Reducing the Risk of Hypoglycemia

Low blood glucose reactions are not always preventable, but there are things you can do to keep them to a minimum.

- Eat meals and snacks on time. A delay of half an hour or more can result in hypoglycemia.
- Make sure that the proper insulin dose is prepared and given. Children require close supervision with this task.
- Plan for extra activity with extra food or an insulin reduction. Set up a good communication system with teachers, coaches, and other leaders so you'll know when extra activity is planned.
- Negotiate realistic blood glucose targets with your health

care team. For example, it may be inappropriate and even dangerous to aim for "normal" blood glucose levels in very young children.

- Remember to lower the insulin dose if the glucose level is low at the same time of day two days in a row, or twice in a week.
- Always have some form of quick-acting glucose close by— and make sure everyone knows where it is.
- Make sure that teens are aware that drinking alcohol can cause delayed hypoglycemia.
- Always have a glucagon kit at home. Review its use regularly. Take it with you on vacation. Replace it when it reaches its expiry date, and practice preparing it before you throw it out.
- Encourage your child to wear medical-alert identification, and to carry a wallet card if older.

False Low Blood Glucose Reactions

Sometimes children feel anxious, nervous, or tired and think it's due to low blood glucose when it isn't. There are many reasons for this. A quick blood glucose check is the best way to find out whether or not the blood glucose is low. Sometimes low blood glucose symptoms occur when the blood glucose drops quickly from a high to a normal level. Feeling nervous or upset for other reasons, such as exams, can also be confused with hypoglycemia. And occasionally the symptoms of high blood glucose are mistaken for a low glucose reaction. Once the blood glucose has been checked and it is clear that the result is not low, reassure the child that he or she can resume the activity. However, if in doubt, treat the symptoms.

High Blood Glucose (Hyperglycemia)

Parents of children with diabetes quickly discover that, no matter how much they know about the disease, and no matter how hard they try to get excellent blood glucose results, the levels will be high from time to time. This is to be expected. Sometimes the reasons are obvious—a test done too soon after the last meal or snack, a lazy rainy day, an extra treat at a birthday party, or some insulin leakage from an injection site. Sometimes the reason is less obvious like a bottle of insulin that was inadvertently frozen, heated, or ruined in some other way, and which requires that you open a fresh bottle of insulin. Often, however, there's no obvious reason for the high level, which will seem unfair to those who invest a lot of time and effort in controlling blood glucose. But it's no one's fault. Rather it's the result of an imperfect means of replacing insulin. Injecting insulin even three or four times a day does not restore the automatic blood glucose regulation that people without diabetes take for granted. There will be occasional highs regardless of how careful you are.

Blood glucose results on their own do not tell the whole story. Parents should also want to know if their child:

- is experiencing any symptoms of hyperglycemia, such as thirst, increased urination, or fatigue
- is showing signs of being sick, such as a cough or fever
- has ketones in the urine or blood

An isolated high blood glucose level—even one in the high teens or twenties (300–400 mg/dL)—is no cause for concern as long as the child feels well and there are no ketones in the urine. If high blood glucose levels persist, even in the absence of symptoms or ketones, an insulin adjustment may be required. (See Chapter Five.)

A high blood glucose level combined with ketones in the

blood or urine or with the signs and symptoms of high blood glucose such as increased urination and thirst, indicates a need for immediate action. Additional short-acting or rapid-acting insulin (regular, NovoRapid, or Humalog) should be injected. The diabetes team will help you decide how much insulin to give. Failure to take action when the blood glucose level is high and ketones are present can lead to diabetic ketoacidosis, a life-threatening condition.

High Blood Glucose Symptoms
- urinating more than usual (polyuria)
- getting up in the night to urinate (nocturia)
- bedwetting (enuresis)
- thirst (polydipsia)
- poor energy level, tired, and irritable (and doesn't get better with food)
- blurred vision
- weight loss

Diabetic Ketoacidosis (DKA)

DKA is a serious situation that develops when there is a lack of insulin in the body. This may occur at the time of diagnosis (some 10 to 25 percent of children with newly diagnosed diabetes have arrived in the emergency room with DKA) or if one of three situations arises:
- failure to get any or enough insulin
- failure to take sufficient extra insulin to cover the high glucose and ketone production caused by infection or other illness
- For those on insulin pumps—undetected or inappropriately managed pump failure

With insufficient insulin available, blood glucose levels rise and excess glucose spills into the urine. Then the body starts breaking down fat as an alternative supply of energy, and the child gets tired and starts to urinate and drink a lot. The ketones produced by fat breakdown are acidic, causing ketoacidosis. As more and more water is lost in the urine and as vomiting occurs with DKA, severe dehydration results. DKA can be avoided as long as the child gets all of the insulin all of the time and as long as illnesses are managed appropriately.

DKA usually develops over hours or days. For those using insulin pumps DKA can happen more quickly than for those on a combination of rapid- and intermediate- and long-acting insulin injections. This is because children on pumps use rapid-acting insulin only and there is no background insulin in their system. Symptoms include:

- high blood glucose levels and ketones in the urine or blood
- excessive thirst
- urinating much more often and in larger amounts
- sudden loss of weight
- complaints of stomach pains or nausea
- vomiting
- leg cramps
- a flushed appearance
- headache
- signs of dehydration: dry mouth and tongue, sore throat, dark circles under the eyes
- deep, heavy breathing, fruity-smelling breath
- drowsiness leading in time to unconsciousness

If a child exhibits any of these signs, the blood glucose level should be checked along with the presence of urinary ketones. Notify the doctor right away. DKA must be treated in a hospital.

Preventing DKA

Since one of the main reasons for developing DKA is failure to get enough insulin, clearly parents need to ensure that children and teens are getting the right amount of insulin at the right time. This responsibility is too much for a young child to assume alone. The other high-risk time for developing DKA is when the body is under stress due to fever—infection or flu, for example. These common conditions can become life-threatening if they are not adequately managed by the family with the support of their health care team. Become very familiar with the sick-day guidelines that follow, and remember—if you're taking a vacation, don't leave home without them.

Sick Days

Children with diabetes do not experience more illnesses than their non-diabetic friends, and they should not miss more school days just because of their diabetes. An otherwise healthy person with well-controlled diabetes has normal resistance to infection. When diabetes is adequately controlled, injuries are not slow to heal. However, while illness may not be more likely, or more difficult to treat in a person with diabetes, any illness may upset the blood glucose balance.

When children with diabetes get sick, their blood glucose often goes high and ketones may show in the urine or blood. Illness is a stress to the body, and stress creates a demand for more insulin. People without diabetes automatically make more insulin at such times. Children with diabetes do not. So on a sick day the usual amount of insulin may not be enough, and monitoring may show high blood glucose, with or without ketones. At such times you may need to increase the insulin dose, even though the appetite may be poor, to prevent DKA.

Although all illnesses in people with diabetes must be taken seriously, not all illnesses make the blood glucose go up. In fact, illnesses like diarrhea may be accompanied by low blood glucose levels. Careful monitoring of blood glucose levels and urinary or blood ketones will help determine the effect of each illness and the appropriate response.

What to Do When a Child with Diabetes Is Ill

- Check the blood glucose and urinary or blood ketone levels when the illness first appears (a mild case of the sniffles doesn't warrant checking, but a more severe cold or cough does) and continue to check every 4 hours around the clock.
- Continue administering insulin. Even though the child may not be eating well, the physical stress of the illness will probably raise the blood glucose level and cause ketones to form. Thus more insulin may be needed, rather than less. If the glucose levels go lower, less (but never no) insulin may be required. Remember that insulin is always required to prevent the breakdown of body fat into ketones.
- If the child doesn't want to eat, give clear fluids containing glucose. Offer frequent small amounts of fruit juice, frozen ice treats, glucose-containing fruit-flavored gelatine, or soft drinks.
- Teens with diabetes who are doing their own monitoring and insulin administration should be helped or supervised carefully throughout the illness.
- Be sure to treat the underlying illness that is upsetting diabetes control. Give the medications prescribed. Acetaminophen in the usual doses for fever or pain is safe unless the doctor says otherwise.
- *Telephone the diabetes doctor or nurse immediately* if illness is accompanied by:
    - vomiting
    - eating or drinking poorly
    - urinary or blood ketones

Note: Take vomiting seriously. If the child vomits twice or more within 12 hours, call the diabetes team or take the child to the hospital immediately. Where vomiting is concerned, it is better to overreact than underreact. Continued vomiting may lead to DKA or severe hypoglycemia.

Fluid Guidelines for Sick Days

When a child with diabetes is sick, he or she may be unable to eat the usual amounts of food in the meal plan. It's important to replace the uneaten food with fluids that provide enough glucose to balance the insulin administered.

If the child is on a meal plan and is carbohydrate-counting, provide drinks that contain the right amount of carbohydrate for each meal and snack. It's not necessary for the child to take all the fluid at once; if necessary, the drinks can be spread through the day. For example, if the child is scheduled to have 42 grams of carbohydrate at breakfast and 15 grams as a morning snack, you can provide 10 to 15 grams each hour throughout the morning.

If the child is not carbohydrate-counting, you can provide one of the following choices every hour; each contains 10 grams of carbohydrate:

- half a cup of juice
- one cup of soup
- one-third can of regular ginger ale
- half a Popsicle
- a quarter-cup of regular Jell-O

Insulin Management during Illness

When children are sick they still need insulin at their usual times. In fact, they may require extra injections of short-acting or rapid-acting insulin as often as every 4 hours, if they show high blood glucose and urine or blood ketones. To decide how much insulin to give, check the blood glucose and urine or blood ketones every 4 hours and consult this chart each time. The following illness scenarios offer courses of action depending on results of the blood glucose and urinary or blood ketone results.

Table 6.1 Check Blood Sugar and Ketone Levels Every 2-4 Hours, Consult This Chart, and Take the Recommended Action.

Blood Glucose	Urine Ketones	Blood Ketones	Action
Less than 6 mmol/L (110 mg/dL)	Negative or positive	0–3 mmol/L	If it is time to give insulin, reduce the dose by 10 to 20%. Encourage consumption of glucose-containing fluids. Speak to your doctor if further reductions are required, if your child will not drink, or if vomiting occurs. Be prepared to give mini dose glucagon (see text).
6–14 mmol/L (110–250 mg/dL)	Negative or positive (any amount)	0–3 mmol/L	Give the usual insulin at the usual time, but do NOT give extra. Test again in 4 hours.
Greater than 14 mmol/L (over 250 mg/dL)	Negative or small (+)	0–0.6 mmol/L	Give extra rapid-acting insulin now—up to 10% of the total daily dose. This is given in addition to the usual insulin at the usual time. Test again in 4 hours.
Greater than 14 mmol/L (over 250 mg/dL)	Moderate or large (+, ++)	0.7–3 mmol/L	Give extra short-acting or rapid-acting insulin NOW. At least 10–20% of the total daily dose. This is given in addition to the usual insulin at the usual time. Test again in 4 hours.

To figure out how much more rapid-acting insulin to give, add up the total daily insulin dose. For example, someone taking 20 units of intermediate-acting and 4 units of rapid-acting insulin before breakfast, 4 units of rapid-acting insulin before supper and 7 units of intermediate-acting insulin before bed has a total daily dose of 35 units. Ten percent of 35 units is 3.5 units; 20 percent of 35 units is 7 units, so it is safe to give an extra 4 to 7 units of rapid-acting insulin. For children and teens on pumps, the total daily insulin dose can be found in the memory of the pump. As a general rule, it is wise to check with your doctor or nurse before giving more than 10 additional units at a time. Small children and children who have been diagnosed in the last six months to a year tend to be sensitive to insulin. In this situation you may want to choose a dose at the lower end of the range to start with and then go by your experience.

Sick Day Insulin Dose Adjustment Guidelines for Children on Pumps

Pump users—just like those who receive insulin by injection—will have to take extra care during periods of illness to ensure that neither hypoglycemia nor DKA develops. The following are rules to be followed by pump users during illness.

1. Check blood glucose and urinary or blood ketones immediately and every 2 to 4 hours around the clock. After each check consult the insulin dose adjustment guidelines in Table 6.1 to figure out what to do.
2. During illness the usual correction doses may not be enough. The dose adjustment guidelines in Table 6.1 suggest a correction of 10 to 20 percent of the total daily dose or TDD. For you this means basal plus bolus, a number that can be found in the memory of your pump (i.e., daily totals).

3. When an illness makes the blood sugar go high, increase the basal rate temporarily by 20 percent. Further increases may need to be made depending on the result.

4. A vomiting illness with a high blood glucose level and ketones must be treated as a pump failure until proven otherwise. The big worry here is impending DKA. In this situation, discontinue the pump immediately and use the pen or syringe to inject rapid-acting insulin in the amount of 10 to 20 percent of the total daily insulin (i.e., basal plus bolus). Do not use the pump until mechanical problems have been ruled out and a full set change has been done. Remember, if the pump fails to give insulin, children may get high blood glucose levels and DKA more quickly (a few hours) since they have no background insulin (e.g., NPH, Lantus, Levemir) in their system.

Caution!

A vomiting illness with high sugar and ketones must be treated as a pump failure. Disconnect the pump and give rapid acting insulin immediately with a syringe or a pen. Contact your diabetes nurse or doctor immediately.

Important note: When the blood sugar is high and you give the recommended correction through the pump you should see an effect. If the blood glucose does not go down by at least 3 mmol/L (55 mg/dL) in a 60-minute period when there has been no carbohydrate intake, give the correction bolus with a pen or a syringe and change the infusion set and site.

Mini Dose Glucagon

Sometimes when children are sick they are unable or unwilling to drink and their blood glucose begins to drop very low.

The guidelines that follow provide you with a way to respond to low blood glucose levels when your child is sick and unable to take glucose by mouth. By being prepared to inject tiny doses of glucagon at home when this situation occurs you may be able to avoid an emergency room visit. Mini dose glucagon increases the blood glucose level quite quickly and its action is brief. The dose may have to be repeated.

When to Use Mini Dose Glucagon

You can safely inject your child with a small amount of glucagon if he is sick and the blood glucose levels are persistently under 4–6 mmol/L (70–110 mg/dL) and he is vomiting or cannot take enough glucose by mouth to keep the blood glucose levels above 6 mmol/L (110 mg/dL).

How to Use Mini Dose Glucagon

- prepare the glucagon solution according to the manufacturer's instructions; leaving the mixed glucagon in the vial
- the total volume of the prepared solution is 1 mL, which looks like 100 units of solution in an insulin syringe
- use an insulin syringe to measure the tiny dose of glucagon and inject it in the same way and in the place that you inject insulin
- keep the unused portion of the glucagon solution in the refrigerator for up to 24 hours

How Much Glucagon to Use for Sick Days

- The dose of glucagon depends on the size and the child and how well she responds.
- If your child is less than 2 years old, inject 2 units of glucagon.
- For children aged 2 to 15 years, give 1 unit of glucagon per year of age. The maximum dose is 15 units. For example if the child is 4 years old, the dose of glucagon is 4 units. If the child is 17 years old, give 15 units of glucagon—the maximum dose.

- If the blood glucose is still low (under 4–6 mmol/L or 70–110 mg/dL) 30 to 60 minutes after injecting the glucagon, you may repeat the glucagon but this time double the dose. For example the 4-year-old child who took 4 units the first time should have 8 units on a repeat dose. Remember the maximum dose is 15 units.
- Check the blood glucose at least every 30 minutes until the blood glucose is over 6 mmol/L (110 mg/dL) and then hourly until the child is able to take enough glucose by mouth to keep the blood glucose level in a safe range.
- Mini dose glucagon should not be given more than five times in a 24-hour period.

Caution: If your child is vomiting repeatedly (for example, two to three times within 1 or 2 hours) or is dehydrated—dry sticky mouth and sunken eyes—do not use the glucagon. In this case it is safer to take your child to the closest emergency room for assessment and treatment.

Surgery
Most operations do not present problems for someone with diabetes, as long as careful attention is paid to blood glucose control before, during, and after surgery.

Surgery under local anesthesia usually does not require hospital admission. However, it is important that meals not be missed. Dentists, for example, should be told about the diabetes, and appointments for tooth extraction or root canal work should be scheduled so they don't interfere with meal or snack times.

If surgery under general anesthetic is required, hospital admission may be necessary and a physician experienced in the management of type 1 diabetes should be involved. Admission may be either one day before the surgery or on the day of surgery. On the day of surgery, an intravenous line will be used to supply fluids containing glucose until normal eating resumes. Also, the insulin dosage will be adjusted as necessary.

Q&A

I read that the symptoms of insulin reaction or diabetic ketoacidosis can be confused with drunkenness. Is that true?

It's true. The slurred speech, confusion, staggering, and fatigue of hypoglycemia can look like drunken behavior. DKA may also be mistaken for drunkenness because the breath can smell a bit fruity, which can be confused with the smell of alcohol. However, what happens more often is that a person with diabetes has a couple of drinks, then begins to go low. (Alcohol causes low blood glucose if food isn't eaten at the same time.) A bystander who is unaware of the diabetes may smell alcohol on the breath and decide that the person is drunk. This is another good reason for someone with diabetes to wear a medical-alert bracelet.

My teenage son doesn't like to wear his medical-alert bracelet. How can I convince him it's the right thing to do?

While some children feel self-conscious about labeling themselves as having a special condition, these little medallions can be life-savers. Remind your son that the older he gets, the more time he will spend away from you, and with people who don't necessarily know he has diabetes. He needs to protect himself when you're not there.

Many young people find that wearing a medical-alert bracelet can be an ice-breaker when they are unsure about raising the subject of diabetes. When new friends ask about the bracelet, they have the opportunity to explain, if they choose to do so.

How many insulin reactions are too many?
The occasional mild low blood sugar reaction, perhaps one or two per week, which can be easily treated with juice, is to be expected. However, these mild reactions can interrupt the school day or other activities, and make it difficult for the child to concentrate for the following half-hour or so. Prevent them as best you can, and respond to them quickly. Frequent lows need to be addressed with a change to the regimen. For example, if the teacher notices that your child is cranky every day at 11:30 a.m. and low blood glucose is confirmed, it's time to re-examine the meal plan or insulin dose and make a change.

What are the long-term effects of a severe low?
The greatest long-term effect is the fear that the child will have another severe insulin reaction. This is a very real fear for many parents, siblings, and children with diabetes, and it can cause a reluctance to keep trying to maintain good blood glucose control. This psychological setback is the only real long-term impact, because the body works very hard to protect the brain during events like this. Mildly delayed intellectual development has been noted in infants who experienced repeated episodes of severe hypoglycemia in the first 3 to 5 years of life.

My 14-year-old son has had diabetes for three years. He is now receiving three injections a day of NPH and Humalog. His last A1C was 7.9 percent. He is conscientious and responsible for his own diabetes care but still has low blood glucose reactions at night, two or three times per month. Would a pump help?
Giving insulin by continuous infusion with the pump may indeed reduce the risk of low blood glucose levels in the night, since the pump administers only very tiny amounts of insulin

at a time. You describe your son as responsible and conscientious, both important attributes for pump therapy. To be successful, your son will be asked to become an expert carbohydrate counter and hopefully, with your help, he'll be required to check his blood glucoses more frequently (i.e., before and after meals and in the middle of the night) during the first few weeks of being on the pump. The use of a long-acting "peakless insulin" such as Lantus or Levemir together with a rapid-acting insulin prior to meals may also reduce the risk of low blood glucose levels through the night.

I heard that people sometimes smear honey in the mouth of a person with diabetes who is unable to swallow. Is this okay?
The big risk of giving an unconscious person anything by mouth is that the person may choke on it. Smearing honey on the lips or between the gums and cheek of an unconscious person with diabetes is better than trying to pour juice or force a hard candy into the mouth. But using glucagon is the best way to reverse a severe hypoglycemic episode rapidly.

Is it possible to get diabetic ketoacidosis from eating too much glucose?
No. The worst that can happen is high blood glucose (hyperglycemia), which is undesirable but not the life-threatening condition of DKA. The only cause of DKA is a lack of insulin.

Is it all right to give my child cough syrup and other medicines?
Health Canada suggests that no oral cough/cold medications be given to children under 6 years of age. If your child is older than 6 years and there is a cough syrup you find effective for your child, by all means use it as directed. The glucose content

of the prescribed dose is probably minimal. However, if you're worried about the glucose in medications, ask your pharmacist to suggest preparations that are glucose-free.

Children with diabetes don't require medicine more often than other children. However, if the doctor prescribes a course of antibiotics, for example, it's important to finish out the prescription, even if blood glucose levels begin to rise. Many parents mistakenly think the antibiotics are the cause of the blood glucose increase, but in fact the illness is probably causing stress on the body, leading to higher glucose levels.

There are medications containing steroids such as prednisone, sometimes prescribed for children with asthma, that actually do cause blood glucose to rise. These drugs can create a need for much more insulin, but they should not be withheld if they're needed. Be prepared to increase the insulin dose.

Should my child have a flu shot every year?
Children with diabetes do not get flu any more frequently or severely than their non-diabetic friends. However, when they do get sick the diabetes may be affected, as discussed. Having a flu shot may prevent your child from missing a few days of school and a period of upset in diabetes control. Children with diabetes should have the flu shot and all the other recommended immunizations.

Older children can treat mild reactions with dextrose tablets or hard candies. What would you suggest for infants and toddlers?
Clearly hard candies and dextrose tablets are inappropriate for young children. Three or four ounces (90–125 mL) of juice in a bottle or cup would work. Also, some parents keep a tube of cake frosting handy for treating mild hypoglycemia.

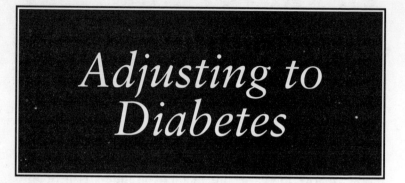

SEVEN

Adjusting to Diabetes

❝ Sometimes my folks and I seem to come from different planets," says Melissa, a 14-year-old who has had diabetes for the past eight years. "They seem to care only about my blood glucose numbers and not how I feel about myself. They don't trust me to take care of myself."

Melissa's parents see it another way. "Melissa's a great kid, but left to her own devices, we're worried that she wouldn't test her glucoses and might even skip a few insulin shots," says her mother, Joan. "It's so hard to let go after doing everything for her all these years, and she's not mature enough to make the right decisions on her own."

Melissa's situation is common among teenagers with diabetes. The struggle for independence versus the parents' reluctance to give up their caretaking role is one of the many phases of dealing with diabetes. From the day of diagnosis, diabetes has an immediate impact on the psychological, emotional, and social functioning of the young person, as well as the family. Through the years, as the child or teen matures, the family faces many emotional challenges.

Dealing with the Diagnosis

The diagnosis of diabetes elicits many reactions in both child and parents. Most children and their families go through a grieving period at first and experience a variety of feelings that may include shock, denial, sadness, anxiety, fear, anger, and guilt. Over time, families do adjust and get on with life as they knew it; they find themselves adapting and readapting to diabetes, and feeling some of these emotions again and again.

Shock or Denial

"This can't be true!" When we experience a crisis our first reaction is often one of shock. This is our body's way of cushioning the blow. It's natural to feel numb and, early on, parents often say the reality hasn't hit them yet. Others describe the feeling as a bad dream from which they keep hoping to wake up. This feeling of shock is usually short-lived.

Sadness

"It feels like this is the end of the world." When we grieve, we feel a sense of loss or a deep sadness. Parents can feel shattered by the knowledge that their child has to receive injections, do blood tests, and stick to a meal plan, and that these changes are likely permanent. Parents and children may mourn their old way of life. Children may be upset that they can't eat whatever and whenever they want to, or worry that it will affect their activities and friendships. Parents may feel bad that they have to say no sometimes to even healthy food because it isn't the right time of day to eat. Experiencing these emotions may help us begin to redefine our lives and put the pieces back together. Once people have expressed their sadness and sense of loss, they start to see the many parts of their lives, and the many hopes for their future, that don't have to change.

Fear and Anxiety

"How will we ever cope?" Confronted with diabetes and its implications, parents feel anxious about their child's health. Some worry about their ability to juggle the complex tasks required for good diabetes management, while others are more concerned about low blood glucose reactions. Some feel stressed about having to give injections or finger pricks. Still others worry about their child's future health, and wonder whether she will be able to manage alone in later years. Some children fear needle pricks or finger pricks in the beginning, and younger children, when they see their parents' distress, may even think they're going to die. However, their fear and anxiety often serve to focus the parents' attention on the needs of their children.

Anger and Resentment

"Why me?" Young people can be angry about developing diabetes. They may hate the injections, blood tests, and food restrictions, and feel their world has turned upside down. They may feel it just isn't fair that they have to deal with this disease and its demands. Parents, too, can feel angry that this has happened, and helpless to change it. They may resent the extra responsibilities forced upon them. But anger can also empower parents in responding to and defending their children's needs.

Guilt

"What did we do wrong?" Parents often wonder if their child's diabetes is due to something they did, or blame themselves because diabetes runs in their family. Some feel guilty because they didn't notice the signs earlier. Children may feel they are burdening their parents. Some feel guilty, believing they must have done something wrong to cause the diabetes. There is absolutely no reason to feel guilty; there is nothing anyone can do to cause or prevent type 1 diabetes. Guilt can be managed by refocusing on the things we do have some control over, such as treatment and future health.

All these difficult emotions can turn out to be positive and protective forces. But they can also be detrimental, if parents or children get stuck in one of these states. Talking about these early emotional reactions, and learning to manage them, helps families move along the path toward adjustment. During these early stages, the support of the diabetes team, including the social worker and psychologist or behavioral specialist, is very important. Their roles are not only to help stabilize the immediate medical condition, but also to provide ongoing support to the child and family.

Living with Diabetes

Adjusting takes time and patience for all family members. Everyone may have to get up a bit earlier on weekdays to accommodate the new routine; children may not be able to sleep in as late on weekends; parents will need to plan meals in advance instead of acting spontaneously (at first, anyway), and will have to remember to pack extra food for the child when he or she leaves the house. In the long run, though, all these adjustments become second nature.

Whenever possible, both parents should be involved in all phases of the diabetes care routines. Feelings of resentment, fatigue, and stress can build up if one parent is burdened with all the planning and responsibility. Parents should work together to prevent burnout by sharing the load and giving each other time away from diabetes duties. They need to plan time together, apart from their child or children, just as they did before. The child will also benefit from growing up in a household where diabetes responsibilities are shared evenly.

In single-parent families, it helps if a member of the extended family or a close friend can participate in the child's care from time to time, or provide relief by babysitting. Take steps, though, to ensure that babysitters and other caregivers know enough to look after a child with diabetes safely. Most diabetes teams will provide appropriate education for people participating in care at this level.

The challenge families face is to fit diabetes into their lifestyles, rather than letting it control their lives. This may require some creative problem-solving, often with help from the diabetes team. A strong support system of grandparents, aunts, uncles, siblings, friends, and even support groups can do a lot to help you deal with the demands of diabetes, be it through practical or emotional support. Don't hesitate to ask for help from your diabetes team.

Attitudes and Beliefs

How families cope with diabetes depends to some extent on their attitudes and beliefs. Those who see it as a serious but manageable condition will cope better than those who remain overwhelmed, doubtful of their ability, or negative about the potential long-term consequences of the disease. These attitudes and beliefs may be influenced by the family's prior experience with diabetes. Those who know someone having a difficult time, or experiencing serious complications, may feel very pessimistic about their own future. In this case, the diabetes team can help the family maintain perspective: science and technology have changed the outlook for people with this disorder, and there are positive steps you can take to decrease the chance of complications in later life.

Some parents view their child with diabetes as being sick or fragile at first. With a little time, education, and experience they soon learn that their child is still healthy. They have to resist the urge to be overly concerned and overprotective, as this may interfere with the child's normal development. Diabetes should not stop children and teens from doing all the things their friends would do. It's just that extra planning is needed to ensure their safety.

Balancing Supervision with Independence

Diabetes requires that both the young person and the parents acquire new skills and take on new tasks. These added responsibilities inevitably alter family relationships. With very young children, total responsibility for all aspects of day-to-day activities will fall squarely on the parents. However, as the child grows and matures there will be a slow and steady shift from completely parent-oriented care, through stages of shared care, to complete independence of the late adolescent and young adult in all aspects of diabetes management.

The transfer of responsibility must not be too rapid. New responsibilities should be added only as the child or teen demonstrates competence with those parts of the treatment plan for which he or she is already responsible. The teens who run into the most difficulty with their diabetes are those for whom parental support is either lacking or inconsistent. Some health care providers mistakenly encourage families to give as much responsibility as possible to the child. After all, they argue, it's the child's diabetes and the child must become proficient in its management. The best balance, however, requires that parents continue to support and encourage their teens, to help them achieve and maintain the best possible level of glucose control. Parents obviously walk a thin line between giving too much responsibility too early and being overprotective. That's another reason the diabetes team is there to guide them.

Even when a young teen has been responsible for a good deal of diabetes care without much supervision, the parents will need to become more involved when the going gets tough, such as during periods of illness, stress at school, or other emotional crises.

Emotional Impact on Brothers and Sisters

Siblings go through the same emotions as other family members: guilt that their brother or sister has diabetes and they haven't; fear that they too may get the disease, or that their sibling may become really sick; anger that Mom or Dad stopped buying glucose-coated cereals or baking chocolate chip muffins; jealousy because their sibling seems to get all the attention. It's a challenge, especially at the time of diagnosis, to balance everyone's needs. Brothers and sisters need to be given the opportunity to express their feelings and emotions, and to know that they are still loved. They should be encouraged to participate in the education program, both to involve them in the new family reality and to provide information that will allow them to feel safe and comfortable with their sibling with diabetes. Many parents find that spending "special time" alone with non-diabetic siblings eases the emotional impact on them.

Financial Concerns

The ongoing cost of diabetes supplies can be a concern. The child requires insulin, syringes or insulin pens and needles, or a pump and supplies; blood glucose monitoring equipment (meters and strips); urine test strips; glucagon emergency kits;

and glucose tablets for low glucose reactions. Clearly diabetes is an expensive disease: for example, blood glucose test strips cost eighty cents to a dollar (both U.S. and Canadian) each. For someone checking blood glucose levels four or more times a day, this can add up to a considerable amount of money every year, for the strips alone.

Most extended health or private drug plans cover the cost of most diabetes supplies. For those who have no coverage and cannot afford these supplies, federal or provincial/state plans may help alleviate the burden. Volunteer agencies may also provide financial support. But some families have to pay for diabetes supplies themselves, because they don't have private insurance and they aren't eligible for government plans. This can be quite a hefty load. At the very least, these expenses should be eligible for a medical expense tax credit. If you're in this position, ask your diabetes team about agencies, resources, and strategies that may help ease the financial load.

Impact of the Family and Child on the Diabetes

Just as diabetes impacts on the family, so the way the family functions affects diabetes management. A healthy adjustment tends to be associated with family sharing of responsibilities, feelings of family togetherness, the ability to problem-solve, little conflict between family members, and consistent parenting. When there is overwhelming stress in the family, it's hard to think through problems and solve them effectively. As a result, diabetes care may be compromised.

Healthy attitudes in the parents are key to helping children adjust; children take their cues from their parents and are sensitive to their feelings. When parents are consistent in their expectations and agree on the approach to diabetes management, the child is more likely to comply with routines. It also helps if parents are used to problem-solving and have developed coping strategies around stress in their own lives.

Diabetes and Friends

Childhood and adolescence are periods of frequent and intense social interaction. While parents are trying to figure out how to deal with daily diabetes management, young people are often more worried about how to incorporate this new reality into their lives. Plenty of questions arise: What do I tell my friends? How do I tell them? Will they treat me differently now that I have to take daily injections, check my blood glucose, and eat my meals at specific times? Just as each family has different ways of coping with diabetes in general, children and teens have different styles of telling their friends.

With a little encouragement, most children will choose an open, matter-of-fact approach. Some make a presentation on diabetes to the class as part of show-and-tell. Others choose to share their experience and knowledge as part of a speech or science project. Most classmates are curious, and full of admiration for a friend who is brave enough to endure daily injections and finger pricks.

But not all children are comfortable with this approach. Some hesitate to discuss their diabetes with classmates they hardly know. Rather, they prefer to share the information only with school personnel and their closest friends, the ones they rely on for support. For safety's sake, the families of the child's friends should also be aware of the diabetes, the need for routines, and even the signs and symptoms of a low blood glucose reaction.

Hiding diabetes is not only unsafe, it may be psychologically unhealthy, reflecting unresolved denial or shame. A child who is not prepared to tell friends about his or her diabetes may have poor self-esteem and a lack of confidence. While respecting the child's wish for privacy, parents may have to help the child share the diagnosis with close friends, key school personnel, and other caregivers to ensure a safe environment.

One reason children want to avoid telling their friends is the fear of teasing or shunning. Fortunately, teasing is not that common. If teasing is an issue, children may need some special tips and support in handling the situation.

The family, the school, and the diabetes team can all play a supportive role in helping the child talk to friends and deal with their varied reactions. Parents can speak to the friends' parents and help the child feel more self-confident. The school can explain to classmates that diabetes is not contagious, and that the child with diabetes is no different from other children and can continue to enjoy the same games and activities as before. Among the members of the diabetes team, the social worker or counselor is usually best equipped to deal with these coping issues, recognizing children's varied backgrounds, personal experiences, and family dynamics.

Strategies for Adjustment

In addition to the usual varied stresses most families face, families living with diabetes face additional demands. How can they ease the burden and adjust to the disease as smoothly as possible?

- Learn as much as possible about diabetes. Becoming an expert means you'll more likely be ready when a challenge arises.
- Keep in regular contact with the diabetes team. These health professionals are there to help with problem-solving. Sometimes a call to one of the team can quickly solve a problem that seems insurmountable. Don't let a small problem grow.

- Explore community and social supports. Knowing other families who have a child with diabetes, belonging to a parent support group or, for teens themselves, joining a diabetes youth group may lessen the tension by providing the opportunity to meet understanding peers.
- Share the responsibility. In two-parent families, find an appropriate balance of responsibilities and activities related to diabetes care. Single parents should try to find a support person who is willing to learn the basics about the child's diabetes routines and to provide necessary relief. With this backup in place, the child remains safe when the parent is not available.
- Remember what worked before to relieve stress. Fall back on familiar ways of coping that have worked in the past. This may involve taking time out, going for a walk, talking with a friend, listening to music, or enjoying a vigorous physical workout.
- Manage feelings—don't hide them. Although it is often hard for parents to see their children upset, it is important to allow them to express painful feelings about having diabetes. This helps children feel understood and supported, and parents feel relieved knowing what the problem is. Solid communication builds trust and promotes problem-solving, important factors in healthy adjustment to a chronic disorder.
- Use distractions. For the small child, in particular, the actual performance of blood glucose checks and insulin injections may cause tension. Have the child hold a teddy bear during the injection, perform the finger pricks while the child watches television, or have a sibling sit with the child while the routines are completed.
- Try not to focus only on the diabetes. Remember that children lead busy and active lives. Make an effort to focus on

their schoolwork, their friends, or their extracurricular activities. Get involved in these activities in a way that's consistent with your lifestyle, and demonstrate by your action and interest that diabetes is not your only shared activity.

- Avoid black-and-white thinking. Diabetes care can be complicated, and it's important not to think of outcomes as good or bad. Blood glucose and A1C levels should be thought of as high or low, not good or bad. Furthermore, diabetes care is not an all or nothing issue. Viewing temporary problems as slips, not failures, will make adapting easier.

Diabetes in the Classroom

The demands of diabetes management cannot help but have an impact on school life. School personnel must be aware of the student with diabetes. By understanding the important aspects of diabetes management, the teacher can ensure the student's healthy adjustment to the classroom setting and peer interactions. Teachers also play an important part in ensuring the safety of the student with diabetes, not only in the classroom but in the playground, on school trips, and in sports activities. A knowledgeable and supportive teacher will help allay parental anxiety, and will prevent minor crises from getting out of hand. A poorly informed or misinformed teacher who has great anxiety about having a student with diabetes in the classroom can add to the adjustment and management difficulties encountered by the child and the family.

To avert potential problems, arrange a meeting with the child's teachers and other school personnel at the beginning of the school year (or soon after diagnosis, if that happens during the school year) to discuss the child's individual needs. Give them the appropriate information about your child's diabetes. If you complete an information form (on page 157), it may help them remember important facts about your child's needs.

General health care is the responsibility of the family, with the help of the diabetes team. Teachers and other school personnel (excluding the school nurse) are not health care professionals, but they do have a role to play in supporting students and ensuring their safety. It is unrealistic to expect the majority of teachers to be well informed about every disorder that a student may someday show up with. However, when a student with a disorder does arrive in their classroom, teachers and school personnel should gain the necessary know-how to provide support. How much participation is expected from teachers will depend on the child's age, stage of development, and diabetes routines.

The most important thing for teachers to know about diabetes is how to recognize hypoglycemia and prevent a mild insulin reaction from escalating into a more severe one. Teachers of younger children need to be especially observant during gym periods and remind the child with diabetes to take a snack. Teachers should also understand that meal plans are an important element of diabetes care, and that it's hard for children with diabetes to participate in surprise pizza parties or snacks. Teachers should inform parents of any such events so the child's meal plan and insulin dose can be adjusted accordingly. They should be aware of the need for between-meal snacks. Similarly, they should become familiar with the signs of hyperglycemia, and notify parents if the child has to leave the classroom to go to the bathroom more frequently than usual.

In general, teachers should not be expected or required to perform blood glucose checks, give an insulin injection, or operate an insulin pump. However, school personnel should understand enough about the procedures that they will allow the child privacy to do injections and blood glucose testing,

Keeping the School Informed

When completed, this form contains the information parents need to provide to teachers and school personnel at the beginning of each school year. The information should be updated as necessary.

Student's name _____ Age _____ Grade _____

Parents' names _____

Address _____

Phone: home _____ Business _____ Cell/pager _____

Alternate person to call in an emergency _____

Phone_____

Are there siblings in school?   Yes _____ No _____

   Names _____ Grades _____

Doctor's name _____ Phone _____

Health insurance number_____

Time(s) of day when an insulin (hypoglycemic) reaction may occur:

_____

Symptoms commonly experienced by the student: _____

_____

What has been provided to treat the reactions:_____

_____

Where is this sugar source located? _____

   alternatives   4 oz (125 mL) fruit juice
                      4 oz (125 mL) regular soft drink (not diet)

Type of morning snack_____

Type of afternoon snack_____

Suggested treats for in-school parties _____

Suggested food for extra activities _____

Special instructions _____

_____

_____

_____

_____

_____

_____

_____

and supply any necessary supervision. The school should have a plan of action in place in case the child has a severe insulin reaction: administer glucose or juice if the child is conscious; if unconscious, call an ambulance. If the child vomits, the parents or some other designated, responsible adult should be notified. If they are unavailable, the teacher must get the child to the nearest emergency room.

Field Trips

Children with diabetes should be encouraged to participate in as many school activities as they choose, and should not be excluded from school trips. However, planning ahead is essential. If they are participating in physical activities beyond those they do on a daily basis, extra food should be packed in their knapsack or lunch box. Include a mix of fast-acting carbohydrate snacks, such as juice boxes and dried fruit to stave off low glucose reactions, and complex carbohydrate snacks such as crackers, breakfast bars, and cookies.

What to Pack on a Field Trip

On field trips of any type, the child with diabetes must have:

- a source of quick-fix concentrated carbohydrate to treat hypoglycemia (i.e., juice boxes, glucose tablets, hard candies)
- visible identification that indicates that the student has diabetes, such as a medical-alert bracelet
- insulin, syringes/pens (or pump supplies) and blood testing equipment, if the trip overlaps a testing or injection time
- an informed adult companion
- the phone number of parents or an alternate, well-informed responsible adult.

Careful preparation for overnight trips or special events will help prevent problems. If the event—for example, a field trip to the zoo—overlaps an insulin injection or blood test time, ensure that one of the teachers or chaperoning parents is taking responsibility for either performing or supervising the task. Children and accompanying adults should always have supplies to treat low blood glucose, such as hard candies, pre-packaged honey, or even a glucagon kit for overnight or longer trips, if a responsible adult is taught how to use it. Children should know how to recognize symptoms of low blood glucose before they are permitted to go on overnight field trips. Before that, look at volunteering as a chaperone yourself.

Summer Camp

For many school-age children and teens, summertime means not only a holiday from school, but also the opportunity to play and spend time with friends at either day camps or overnight residential camps. For children with diabetes the situation is no different, and with proper planning they too can enjoy a fun-filled, healthy, and safe camp experience. The preparation for day camps is similar to preparation for a family day out or a day trip at school. Make sure the child has all meals and snacks prepared and packed. Except for children who are on a lunchtime injection and are able to administer it themselves, with minor adjustments in timing all insulin injections can be given at home as usual. Similarly, at least three daily blood glucose tests can be performed at home, and blood glucose levels can be monitored by a parent. Most children should do a pre-lunch glucose check at camp.

Ask camp staff about the level of activity in which the child will participate. Inform them that the child has diabetes and emphasize the importance of the timing of food intake. The signs and symptoms of hypoglycemia should be explained, and a source of rapid-acting glucose should be supplied to a counselor to treat a low blood glucose reaction. Furthermore, the camp staff must, like teachers, be told what to do in the event of a severe insulin reaction.

What about overnight camps? Are they safe for children with diabetes? Absolutely. However, to provide a happy and safe camping experience and to ensure that the principles of daily diabetes care are followed, the Canadian and American Diabetes Associations and some other organizations have set up camps especially for children with diabetes. Whenever possible, children and teens with diabetes should have the chance to attend such camps. They are usually staffed by doctors and nurses experienced in the care of children with diabetes. In addition, an experienced dietitian is there to assist the children in meal planning. The programming staff are accustomed to working with campers with diabetes, and develop programs to match the timing of daily diabetes routines.

These camps give children the opportunity to spend several days or weeks with other campers who also have diabetes. Having spent most of the school year integrated with children who do not, many campers are excited to be with other campers who are going through the same stages of disease management. Everybody is doing blood checks, testing urine, taking insulin injections, monitoring diet, and watching for low blood glucose reactions. Some children learn to give their own injections for the first time under the direction of the camp nurse and with the encouragement of their summer friends. For others, especially those from smaller communities, this may be their first experience of not being the only child with diabetes.

Children aren't the only ones who benefit from camp. Many parents find comfort in knowing that diabetes routines are being followed and that their children are in the care of competent staff familiar with the disease, whether at the campsite or during multi-day canoe trips. They feel secure in the knowledge that blood glucose checks will be done overnight as necessary, as well as during the day, and that extra snacks will be provided when needed. With such a support system, the children can enjoy the full range of camp experiences, including swimming, boating, tripping, crafts, and drama, without the burden of managing their diabetes care alone.

Some children and teens prefer to go to camps not specifically aimed at those with diabetes. If the child or teen has sufficient knowledge, sense of responsibility, and willingness to monitor the condition, this too can be accommodated by proper planning.

Remember that most children attending camp are more active than usual, and have less access to food between meals. As a result, they may require a lower or different insulin dose to avoid hypoglycemic episodes. More frequent blood glucose monitoring will be needed to determine the actual insulin requirement. Whenever possible, choose a camp with a full-time physician and nurse on site, who can help deal with diabetes routines and any illness that may occur.

Letting Go

The day will come when the child with diabetes is no longer living under the family roof. This transition can be traumatic for both child and parent. No longer will the parent be able to monitor the child's daily log of insulin doses and glucose readings. Nor will the parent be around to pick up on the child's trademark symptoms of an insulin reaction. What is the solution? Start laying a foundation for independence early on. Encourage and support age-appropriate involvement of your child in his or her own diabetes care.

Q&A

Will we ever take a vacation alone again?
It may take a while before you feel comfortable enough with your child's diabetes care to leave someone else in charge. But sooner or later you will. And it's important that you do so, to avoid burnout. You can ease the anxiety by starting off gradually, with a short trip a couple of hours' drive away (you'll feel better knowing you can return home quickly), rather than a two-week vacation in South America. If you know, for example, that you have a week-long business trip you can't miss, you can prepare yourself in advance by spending a night with friends or relatives. Giving a sitter this kind of "dry run" may also alleviate her concerns, as well as the concerns of your child. Give your sitter and any siblings the telephone numbers of your diabetes health care team (and alert the team that they may be called by someone other than yourself). Provide relevant reading material and make up a diabetes care instruction sheet specific to your child.

People keep telling me I should join a diabetes support group, but I'm not sure if they're for me. What are they all about?
Support groups can be invaluable sources of information and advice and, in many cases, new friendships. Your diabetes team or local Canadian Diabetes Association branch can provide names of group leaders. If there is no support group in your area, you may want to start your own. Support groups meet on a regular basis—some follow formal agendas, while others are casual social gatherings. There is little, if any, cost involved, and you're not obligated to attend every meeting. They may be a good place to find babysitters.

Some people resist support groups because they don't like the idea of identifying themselves as "afflicted." But in some ways support groups free you from this label, because everyone there knows the road you are traveling. You don't have to explain the biology and psychology of diabetes to get to the point of your problem. Sharing experiences provides a way to learn more about diabetes, and to feel more secure about your effectiveness in dealing with it.

Every time Billy's grandparents come to visit, they shower him with chocolate and candy. How can we make them see this is harmful for Billy?
It's natural for grandparents to want to give gifts to their grandchildren. You may want to encourage them to pamper Billy in other ways, such as with trips to the movies, or snacks like popcorn or chips. When the gifts are food, help Billy accept them graciously, and then help him work the treat into his meal plan.

Our daughter does well in school but often complains of headaches or stomach cramps due to anxiety about going to school in the morning. What does this mean?
Your daughter may be experiencing school avoidance, which occurs commonly in children with a chronic condition such as diabetes. There are many reasons why children may become anxious. In a child with diabetes, the avoidance may have to do with being teased, or with fear of having a low glucose reaction. Take time to explore your daughter's anxieties about school and diabetes, and seek help from your diabetes team. Ensure that she misses as little school as possible.

The children at my son's school keep teasing him about his diabetes. What should I do?
We can all remember being teased about something at some stage of our childhood—wearing glasses, having skinny legs,

even just bringing something unusual for lunch! Diabetes can be one more target for teasing, but the subject may be a particularly sensitive one, not only for your son but for you as well. It's important to recognize your own vulnerability here, so that you can put the teasing in perspective and work with your son to generate some creative solutions.

An impromptu family discussion about how to handle teasing and the teasers often helps give the child some ideas, as well as moral support. Some children learn to use humor as a response. For others, knowledge is power. It allows them to deal confidently with their classmates' misconceptions, and gains them respect for coping with the disease.

If you believe the teasing results from ignorance, you and your son may want to talk to his teacher about strategies to help his classmates understand the basics of diabetes, and what it means to live with it.

EIGHT

Growth and Development

isa is a typical 12-year-old—being with friends is the most important thing in her life. She and three other girls spend almost every waking hour together, talking about boys, trying new hairstyles, turning cartwheels in the backyard. Lisa likes her friends and cares what they think. They know she has diabetes and she doesn't want them to think for one minute that it means she can't do everything they can. This is a good attitude on Lisa's part, but it could get her into trouble if it prevents her from sticking to her diabetes routines. For instance, one day after school Lisa was so caught up in hanging out with her friends that she forgot she needed to get home for her afternoon snack. By 4:30 she felt shaky, hungry, and a little dizzy. Fortunately one of her friends had a little candy that she gave Lisa, and after a few minutes Lisa felt better. Of course, Lisa's mom was upset when she found out, but she understood Lisa wanting to stay with her friends. So they made a deal: from now on Lisa will always carry an extra snack with her, in case she's going to be late.

Each age and stage of life presents a different set of challenges relating to both physical and emotional growth and development. A chronic disorder brings additional challenges. It seems that, as soon as the family has found ways to negotiate the rocky course of one stage of development, it's time to go to the next stage. For example, parenting a school-age child with diabetes can be much different from parenting an infant or toddler. Likewise, being a teenager with diabetes is different from being 9 or 10 and living with the disorder. As teenagers reach adulthood, they are faced with new issues that further affect their diabetes care.

The family and the diabetes team can both help smooth the road to adulthood by promoting a strong sense of identity and self-worth in the growing child. The best predictor of future behavior is past behavior: a child whose course has been relatively smooth throughout early childhood is quite likely to negotiate adolescence successfully. Also, families that provide age-appropriate support and guidance will no doubt have less disruption to deal with during the teen years.

Infants, Toddlers, and Preschoolers

Type 1 diabetes is less common in preschoolers than in older children and adolescents: less than 1 percent of diabetes is diagnosed in the first year of life, and less than 10 percent before the age of 5. Because diabetes is less common in this age group and because the symptoms are often confused with other minor illnesses, the diagnosis is often missed until the baby is very sick and in severe diabetic ketoacidosis. Once the disease is diagnosed, however, the situation can be corrected quickly and long-term management can begin.

Developmental milestones and patterns affect the very young child's perception of the world. Normal infants and toddlers generally:

- determine thoughts by what they see and hear
- begin to develop a sense of themselves, first by acquiring a trust in their environment as infants, and then by testing this environment in the next few years
- enhance their knowledge of the world around them through constant exploration, language development, and inquiry ("Why this? Why that? Why the other thing?")
- begin to become more curious and self-directed, choosing some activities and rejecting others

Diabetes care in children under 5 involves a balance between what might be considered ideal—close to normal blood glucose readings—and what is safe and practical. The target range for these young children—pre-meal glucoses of 6–12 mmol/L (110–220 mg/dL)—allows good blood glucose control while reducing the risk of severe hypoglycemia. Too tight control in infants and toddlers is especially risky as they cannot yet recognize the symptoms of low blood glucose. Similarly, one must aim to avoid marked elevations in the blood glucose, which may lead to changes in mood and concentration. Repeated episodes of severe hyper- or hypoglycemia in these children may lead to mild intellectual or learning impairment later in life.

Very young children often have fluctuating appetites. They don't always eat the same amount of food from day to day. If pre-meal blood glucose levels are allowed to go slightly higher than those expected for older children, the infant or toddler is more likely to remain safe even during periods of food refusal or picky eating. Parents will be less worried and frustrated and mealtime will be more pleasant. As children grow they become more predictable in their eating, and more able to recognize and describe their low blood glucose reactions. At that time blood glucose targets also change.

Signs of a Healthy Infant or Toddler with Diabetes

How do parents and others who care for young children know that everything is going well? Look for:

- normal growth and weight gain
- developmental milestones, such as rolling over, sitting up, crawling, standing, walking and talking, at about the normal age
- no signs of high blood glucose levels; good energy, not overly wet (diapers) or unusually thirsty
- few mild low blood glucose reactions, and no severe reactions
- no ketones in the urine
- blood glucose readings that are not too low—less than 6 mmol/L (110 mg/dL)
- blood glucose readings that are not too high for long periods of time—over 12 mmol/L (220 mg/dL)
- a happy and secure attitude in the child

Impact of Diabetes on an Infant, Toddler, or Preschooler

Young children with type 1 diabetes progress through the same stages of development as their friends without diabetes. Nevertheless, the routines and tasks needed for good diabetes care may influence and sometimes interfere with this development. All parents of young children with diabetes worry about the effects of diabetes on their growth as individuals, and how they will cope with the condition as they grow older.

Specific areas of concern include:

- the young child's inability to express symptoms of hypoglycemia (e.g., is the toddler having a hypoglycemic spell or a temper tantrum?)
- dealing with their own and their child's anxiety about the pricks and injections

- developing a structured but flexible treatment plan that does not interfere with the child's normal daily activities, including naps
- providing meals and snacks on time and in consistent amounts (toddlers with picky appetites can really cause stress at mealtimes)

Try to balance the child's need for support and protection against the risk of overprotection and exclusion from age-appropriate activities.

Eating habits change rapidly during the first 5 years of life. Some infants and toddlers are relatively consistent in their eating patterns; most, however, have wide fluctuations in appetite and the amount of food they eat. It's important that the diabetes care routine reflect that. For safety's sake, young children should eat at regular meal and snack times—at least three meals and three snacks a day. But beyond that, imposing a highly structured meal plan on an infant or toddler may only heighten the stress in the family, and even interfere with the child's normal development. As the child gets older, more structure in meal planning becomes both possible and necessary.

Coping Strategies

Some helpful hints in coping with diabetes in a young child include:

- Try to adopt a matter-of-fact approach to insulin injections, finger pricks, and mealtimes. Young children quickly pick up on parents' anxieties and use them to manipulate their environment. Try to be quick, calm, and reassuring when carrying out routines. Reduce the child's fears by preparing the insulin or blood testing equipment in another room before involving the child. When it's over, give the child a big hug and a kiss.

- Share responsibility for the routines wherever possible. This prevents the toddler from playing one caregiver off against the other. In single-parent families, have a friend or family member participate in the diabetes routines on a regular basis. The parent, the toddler, and the support person can remain confident that the child will be safe in the parent's absence.
- Acknowledge the child's feelings and provide reassurance, but don't delay needles or finger pricks until the child is "ready." Consider using distractions such as toys, songs, or television.
- Try to allow the child some control over the routine if he or she wishes, for example, choosing the finger for the next prick.
- For the really picky eater, set limits on time allowed for meals and snacks. Don't sit for hours fighting over each morsel of food. The child always wins.

Tommy is 2 1/2, and doing quite well with his diabetes routines. His parents, Heather and Marc, are sharing responsibility for his finger pricks and insulin injections. Heather gives the morning shot and Marc does the second one, before the evening meal. Tommy's 4-year-old brother, Tyler, is usually asleep during Tommy's morning routine—which suits Heather just fine—but Tyler likes to help his dad with the evening blood glucose check and insulin shot, leaving Heather free to get dinner on the table. Meal and snack times are consistent. Both boys enjoy settling in for their morning snack just as their favorite television program starts at 10 a.m. Afternoon snack works equally well, following Tommy's nap, at 3 p.m. The only problem for Heather comes when Tommy sleeps past 3 p.m. She hates to wake him, figuring he must need his sleep, but how long can she safely let him nap? Unlike children without diabetes, he can't nap right through his snack time. She decides, with the help of her diabetes team, that an extra half-hour is the limit.

Lately Tommy has been refusing food, especially at mealtimes. Worried about lows, Heather and Marc have been pleading, coaxing, and even preparing two or three food choices, but in the end Tommy holds out for apple juice. After discussion with the diabetes team, Heather and Marc decide to reduce the insulin dose a little and adjust the blood glucose targets to 8–12 mmol/L (145–220 mg/dL), from 6–12 mmol/L (110–220 mg/dL), to allow for food refusal, and to limit mealtime to a maximum of 25 minutes. They also plan to resist, if possible, replacing the meal with apple juice alone. Food refusal is a temporary stage many toddlers go through. As Tommy's appetite becomes more predictable, they will have to increase the insulin and reset the blood glucose targets.

The School-Aged Child

Starting school is an exciting time for both child and parents. Children will spend a major part of their day away from home, away from the parents' watchful eye. Not until late childhood or early adolescence can the child be expected to understand diabetes treatment fully, and integrate all its important concepts, such as timing and amounts of insulin injections, blood glucose checks, and consistency in eating habits.

Normal developmental patterns in the early school years include:

- learning to solve concrete problems logically
- further development of social skills—the peer group begins to take on more importance
- learning to play by the rules and thrive in a structured and

supportive environment; when children know the rules and can acquire appropriate skills in a fun way, they develop a positive self-image
• learning to conform

Impact of Diabetes on School-Aged Children

Parents usually continue to be the predominant caregivers, but they are more frequently required to share expertise not only with the child but also with other responsible people such as teachers, sports coaches, babysitters, and day care staff.

School-aged children with diabetes may see themselves as different from their peers, which can lead to considerable distress. Classmates may tease them about their needles and finger pricks. Be sure the child has an appropriate understanding of diabetes, but encourage him or her to participate in school and other activities in the same way other children do. Naturally, planning is required, but being excluded from these activities can be detrimental to the child's self-image.

Coping Strategies

• Remain actively involved in all aspects of your child's diabetes care throughout childhood. However, the level and type of your involvement will change as the child participates more and more in the routines. Ongoing parental involvement in a supportive and nonjudgmental manner will help the child overcome hurdles along the way.

• Be prepared for the occasional slip-up. As children assume more responsibility, they make mistakes—eating a little more, skipping a snack, recording a false blood glucose reading, perhaps even missing an injection. These lapses are a normal part of growing up. Expect them and watch for them so you can deal with them before there are any serious consequences. But remember that these lapses are not a sign of failure. Rather, they provide an opportunity to talk about diabetes and its challenges, and to open the door to creative problem-solving.

- Establish routines, such as mealtime and snack time, and stick to these when possible. However, flexibility is key. Don't fret over a change in schedule, but be aware of the adjustments to be made when, for example, a meal or snack is delayed, or an insulin injection is scheduled during a sports event.

- Involve the child in the routines, and acknowledge his or her feelings and concerns about diabetes. Encourage children's mastery of the diabetes routines—choosing snacks, doing finger pricks and insulin injections.

- Children should be encouraged and helped, rather than forced or threatened, to get them to comply with routines. Opt for simple reminders rather than long lectures.

- Try to control your own stresses, frustrations, and anxieties surrounding diabetes. Children are sensitive to these displays and may either mirror your responses, or try to hide things from you to avoid upsetting you. Seek support from the diabetes team, other parents of children with diabetes, or a support group.

Susan is 10 years old and has had diabetes since age 4. Her parents take most of the responsibility for her diabetes but Susan does help out. She has been able to do her own finger pricks and blood checks for a couple of years now, but she must be reminded when to do them. Her parents record the results. Susan is pretty good at choosing the right kinds and amounts of food at mealtimes and snack times. She knows what it feels like to be low, and she knows what to do—take three dextrose tablets. She hasn't yet mastered her insulin injection—she just hasn't been interested, and her parents have been willing to stay in charge. But Susan is in grade five now and her class will be going to an outdoor education camp for three days. Susan is determined to go too. Her parents are anxious and want to say no—but instead, knowing they have several months to prepare, they sit down with Susan and their diabetes nurse and come up with a plan that will prepare the family and the teacher for this adventure.

Because there may not be an adult on the school trip who can prepare and inject insulin safely, Susan's parents agree to work with her over the next few months to ensure that she is confident and competent with insulin injections by the time she's ready to go.

Susan is already able to do her blood glucose and urine ketone checks, so the next step is for her to begin entering results in the logbook for practice one week a month. Susan thinks this is a good idea.

Because she already makes good decisions about food choices every day, Susan's parents will begin to involve her in planning for extra activity with extra food.

Finally, Susan's mother will contact those at the school in charge of organizing the outdoor camp to find out about adult supervision, the program of activity, the meal schedule, and opportunities for communication between Susan and her parents during camp. She will also organize an education session with the adult taking primary responsibility for Susan at camp. This person must remind Susan about testing and insulin injection times, supervise these routines, and, if necessary, help her respond to low blood glucose or get in touch with her family. These are not unrealistic expectations of an adult supervisor of a grade five student.

Adolescence

Adolescence is a time of rapid biological change, accompanied by increasing physical, cognitive, and emotional maturity. It is a time of increasing peer conformity, experimentation, limit-testing, and independence from family. Self-image changes with the emergence of sexuality, and the experience may be difficult and even frightening for some. Diabetes can affect these processes in different ways.

With or without diabetes, the progression of adolescent development varies greatly both across and within age groups, and within individuals. An important milestone is the acquisition of abstract reasoning, which allows the adolescent to understand fully the implications of diabetes and its management. There are, however, many compelling and conflicting factors—peer pressure, parties and other social events, part-time jobs, and a busy life in general—that may interfere with the teen's ability to translate this new awareness into good self-care behaviors.

Even though it may seem that these young people should be more responsible, more able to achieve "good" blood glucose control, adolescence is frequently the time when adequate blood glucose control is most difficult.

Impact of Diabetes on Adolescents

Diabetes management requires a degree of responsibility and behavioral control that is uncharacteristic of adolescents. The daily demands of the disease have an impact on the personal and public lives of these teens, affecting important developmental areas including independence, body image, identity, sexuality, responsibility, and self-esteem. Parents worry a lot about the teenage years, and perhaps more so when their teen has diabetes. Yet recent research suggests that most adolescents navigate this period without too much disruption, and that they are, in fact, quite well adjusted.

Coping Strategies

- Remain involved in your child's diabetes care, at some level, right through adolescence. Diabetes management is a heavy burden to carry alone.
- Let go gradually. Make sure your teen is ready, willing, and able to take on the aspects of diabetes management you are ready to give up.
- Praise adolescents freely. There is no danger of giving them an inflated ego, and positive reinforcement will only yield more of the desired behavior.
- Parents, teens, and the diabetes team must all have the same expectations of the teen and of each other. Is everyone aiming for the same blood glucose targets? Can everyone agree on the frequency of blood glucose monitoring? Can everyone agree about who chooses what foods at mealtime? Goals and expectations should be reviewed jointly, on a regular basis, to be sure they're still appropriate.
- All teens hate to be nagged, but most don't mind a little help. Parents can help get the monitoring equipment ready for a check, instead of simply saying, "It's that time again." Similarly, they can offer to keep the log, instead of complaining that they don't know what's going on because the numbers never get into the book.
- Be prepared to get reinvolved as necessary. Even the most self-sufficient teen is going to need backup during particularly stressful periods, such as a crisis in a relationship, an illness, or a time of overwhelming competing priorities. This is not a step backward; it's just evidence of the family working together to ensure that the teen's health is maintained at all times.

• Teens should be encouraged to develop their own relationships with members of their diabetes team. Allow a teen private time with the doctor or nurse at each clinic visit. It's natural for parents to want to stay informed, and to have time to discuss issues and be part of developing the plan for the next phase. However, teens should be able to expect confidentiality in certain aspects of their health care.

Special Considerations in the Teenaged Years

Smoking and drug and alcohol abuse in both teenage boys and girls, and unplanned pregnancies and eating disorders in girls, are recognized hazards. However, teens with diabetes must be fully aware of the problems associated with these behaviors, and the additional risks to their health. The use of alcohol, for example, increases the risk of severe hypoglycemia, and smoking greatly increases the chance of early stroke, heart attack, and other diabetes-related complications. It is impossible to make wise choices without accurate information.

It is also critical for parents to understand that diabetes routines may become a target for risk-taking behavior. Teens may skip meals or blood glucose checks. Some even skip their insulin. If such behavior seriously compromises diabetes control, resulting in poor school attendance, hospitalization (due to diabetic ketoacidosis), or poor growth or weight loss, parents will need to resume giving the injections and doing the blood glucose checks, regardless of the teen's age, until there is evidence that it's safe to allow the teen to manage independently once again.

Smoking and Drug Use

Many teens try cigarettes. Unfortunately, some become regular users. Experimenting with "street drugs" such as marijuana is also not uncommon. Adolescents try out tobacco and drugs for several reasons: peer pressure, risk-taking, and feeling "grown up," relief from stress, or because the family does.

Smoking dramatically increases the risk of serious diabetes-related complications such as eye and kidney disease, early stroke, and heart attacks. It should be avoided at all costs. Parents, coaches, educators, and health care providers should make sure children know the risks of smoking from a very young age, and should do whatever it takes to discourage the habit. For parents, this should mean giving up smoking themselves. Teens who have already started smoking may benefit from a smoking cessation program offered at school or perhaps at an adolescent medicine clinic or public health unit.

Marijuana impairs the judgment required to recognize and acknowledge the signs of low blood glucose. Marijuana use also triggers food cravings and hunger, leading to overeating which can, in turn, cause high blood glucose. The direct effect of other street drugs on blood glucose level is not well known. They may do other damage, and may also contribute to impaired judgment and risk-taking behaviors such as unprotected intercourse.

Alcohol

Drinking alcohol without precautions can lead to hypoglycemia, because alcohol interferes with the liver's natural ability to make glucose and add it to the bloodstream. Furthermore, under the influence of alcohol, a teen may miss the early warning symptoms of hypoglycemia and progress quickly to a severe episode, which might not be recognized by others who have also been drinking, or by those who, smelling alcohol on the teen's breath, presume he or she has "passed out" from being drunk.

As a general rule, it's better to educate teens with diabetes about alcohol use than to forbid it. They should understand that drinking in moderation is acceptable once they reach the legal drinking age, but that excessive alcohol use will put them at risk. They should always wear or carry identification stating that they have diabetes, in case of a hypoglycemic event. They should also learn to eat when they drink, to avoid hypoglycemia.

Contraception

Teens with diabetes sometimes wonder if they will be able to have children. We know that diabetes does not alter the fertility of young men, nor does it interfere with a young woman's ability to become pregnant. However, in order to best ensure a full-term healthy baby, the young woman with diabetes must plan her pregnancy so that she maintains excellent control both prior to conception and throughout the pregnancy.

All sexually active girls require contraception to prevent unplanned pregnancies. Generally speaking, the same options are available to women with diabetes as to those without. Even women who take an oral contraceptive should use a condom to reduce the risk of sexually transmitted infections. Sexually active teens should consider intercourse an extra activity that uses up energy, requiring a carbohydrate snack afterward.

Teens with diabetes should be provided with information about sexuality, contraception, and pregnancy well in advance of needing it. These discussions should take place with members of the diabetes team, and should be confidential.

Eating Disorders

Eating disorders are common among teenage and young adult women, and are much less common among males in the same age group. Researchers believe they stem from an obsession about gaining control in a life they perceive to be out of control. There are many possible causes of this obsession, depending on the individual's experience. People with anorexia nervosa try to regain control by denying themselves food; people with bulimia nervosa try to regain control by excessive overeating (binging), then purging by self-induced vomiting or with the aid of laxatives. These definitions aren't cut and dried—people with one disorder sometimes exhibit characteristics of the other. In the long term, anorexia can lead to severe weight loss and can be fatal. The constant binging and purging of bulimia can result in severe stomach ulcers and can also be fatal.

In teenage and young adult women with type 1 diabetes, disturbances in eating attitudes and behavior are common and persistent. Full-blown eating disorders occur in as many as 10 percent of teenage girls with diabetes, but even milder disturbances can play havoc with blood glucose control.

Some diabetes-related factors may increase the likelihood of an eating disturbance. At the time of diagnosis there has often been weight loss. With insulin therapy this weight is quickly regained. In the vulnerable girl this may trigger dissatisfaction with her body and the desire to be thinner again. Also, meal planning is an integral part of diabetes treatment. Such planning implies a degree of dietary restraint, another trigger to disordered eating. Finally, some girls discover that by skipping or reducing their insulin dose, they can lose glucose in their urine and keep themselves underweight. Although this may be an effective way to control weight, it invariably leads to poor diabetes control and, in the long run, earlier onset of diabetes-related complications.

Warnings Signs of an Eating Disorder
Eating disorders in people with type 1 diabetes can lead to wild, unexplained fluctuations in blood glucose levels, often outside

the safe range. Frequent low glucose reactions (insulin reactions) or high glucose reactions (excessive thirst and urination, perhaps leading to urinary ketones) may be a sign that an eating disorder is complicating diabetes management. Eating disorders can also be marked by:

- a preoccupation with food and weight, beyond what is required in diabetes management
- a stated desire to lose weight beyond what seems appropriate
- requests for dietary change with low-calorie, low-fat, vegetarian, or other diets to lose weight
- binge-eating episodes
- insulin manipulation

What You Can Do to Help

If you know someone with an eating disorder, there are several things you can do to help.

- Express your concern for the person's health, while respecting the need for privacy. Eating disorders are usually a symptom of a greater psychological problem, and the fact that you are there to help will be appreciated.
- Avoid power struggles around food. Forcing someone with an eating disorder to eat will probably make things worse.
- Examine your own attitudes around food and weight. Are you furthering the idea that "thin is in"?
- Talk about more flexible meal plans with your diabetes dietitian. Perhaps the current meal plan is too restrictive, reinforcing the idea that the person with diabetes is different and deprived.
- Avoid commenting on weight, either positively or negatively, as it only serves to emphasize the importance of appearance.
- Express your concern to your diabetes health care team and get support for the person.

Driving

Driving a car requires accurate judgment and a keen sense of responsibility. Young people with diabetes have an additional responsibility to ensure that their blood glucose is in the right range before they get behind the wheel of a car. Low blood glucose can impair judgment, increasing the risk of an accident. Parents should be certain that teens show responsible self-management before permitting them to apply for a driver's license or lending them the family vehicle. Getting a regular driver's license is not generally a problem, as long as blood glucose control is reasonable and there have been no severe episodes of hypoglycemia in the previous year.

Employment

There are countless examples of people with diabetes who have excelled in a broad range of careers—doctors, lawyers, nurses, politicians, professional athletes, psychologists, accountants, researchers, teachers, and engineers, to mention a few. In general, parents and educators find that young people can be coached and counseled to pursue the career that interests them or for which they have an aptitude. However, it is also important to be aware of current limitations. Two questions are often asked of the diabetes team: "Are there jobs that are not available to people with diabetes?" and "Do some employers discriminate against people with diabetes?" The answer to both questions is yes.

A number of organizations have a blanket rule that prevents employment of people with diabetes. Such employment includes jobs that require operation of a commercial vehicle such as a truck or an aircraft, and jobs in some military or police departments. These rules are based on the risk of hypoglycemia while on the job. Before applying for a particular educational or employment opportunity, teens with diabetes should inquire as to their employability in these areas.

Employer discrimination has been documented over many years. There is often a misconception that people with diabetes will attend their jobs less frequently and perform less effectively than their peers. Young job-seekers with diabetes should stress their personal qualifications, abilities, and ambitions to potential employers. They should not withhold information about their diabetes, but rather stress the fact that they can perform as well as others. If they believe they are being treated unfairly, they should seek advice through their advocacy group, such as the Canadian or American Diabetes Association.

Jackie is 14 and has had diabetes since the age of 7. She's proud of the fact that she manages her diabetes independently. She checks her blood glucose three or four times a day, and takes her insulin three times a day. Already she participates in decisions about insulin dose adjustment. Her hemoglobin A1C checks have been consistently in the 7s, indicating excellent blood glucose control. She's happy and involved in school and extracurricular activities.

At a recent clinic visit, the doctor discovered that, on one of the few occasions when Jackie's blood glucose checks were high, she recorded a lower result. When this was pointed out to Jackie she became very tearful. With a little prompting she was able to tell her diabetes nurse that she felt sad and upset because she was looking forward to a youth group trip to Ottawa, and her parents had agreed that she could go if she maintained "good" diabetes control; she believed that they wouldn't let her go if they saw the high blood glucose results. Jackie asked her nurse to help her explain the doctor's discovery and her feelings and concerns to her mother, who was in the waiting room.

Jackie's mom listened to the explanation, and tears welled up in her eyes. She put her arm around her daughter, saying, "Jackie, that's not what your father and I meant by 'good' control. We should have been clearer about what we expected." In fact, all her parents meant was that she should put in a strong effort. Everyone has occasional highs and lows, sometimes for no apparent reason, and Jackie's parents didn't mean to suggest that they expected perfection. The misunderstanding opened up the opportunity for Jackie and her parents to clarify and renegotiate their goals.

Helpful Hints for All Ages

- Get everyone in the family involved. Diabetes care is a partnership between the child and the entire family. Mothers often shoulder a major share of the responsibility, but fathers need to be part of this as well. Talk about your feelings in an open manner. On the other hand, try not to let diabetes become the focus of every family meal or discussion. Also, recruit the support of others—grandparents, camp counselors, teachers, sports coaches. The more they know about your child, the more comfortable you'll feel when they're in charge.

- Set realistic blood glucose targets. Expecting every blood glucose to be, say, 8 mmol/L (145 mg/dL) is unrealistic. In fact, it's impossible! Good diabetes control means balancing all the aspects of your life and lifestyle, not just focusing on blood glucose results.

- Make good use of your diabetes team. Don't be afraid to ask questions. And ask more questions if the answers don't seem to fit. (See more about getting the most out of your diabetes team in Chapter Ten.)

- Take credit for trying, and don't feel bad about mistakes— they're bound to happen. Diabetes is a complex and often frustrating condition. Doing the same thing two days in a row does not always lead to the same results.

- Experiment a little and see what works for you and your child. What you learn in your diabetes education and clinic sessions provides you with an excellent foundation. You've become a mini-expert in diabetes. But you haven't been given every answer to every question. Also, some things work better for some people. Use your knowledge to experiment a little. For example, taking less insulin before a sports game may work better in a particular situation than eating a large amount of extra food.

- Be realistic in your expectations of what responsibility your child will take for the diabetes. Don't expect too much too soon. On the other hand, try not to be overbearing and overprotective.

- Be careful to praise good performance. It's very easy to focus on the negatives. "You're late for your blood glucose check!" "Did you take your insulin yet?" It's also easy to overlook the positives. Rather, praise every little advance, and look for opportunities for ongoing education when things are a little off track.

- Make some time for yourself and your spouse or significant other. Sometimes the diabetes seems to take up every minute of every day, and you feel as if you have no time for the things you have always loved to do—read a book, take a walk, go to a movie. Your child needs you to be in as good shape as he or she is. Have fun for yourself and also for your child.

Q&A

It takes half an hour of bargaining to get my 3-year-old to cooperate during injection time. How can I make this go more smoothly?

It's not unusual for children of all ages to go through periods when they cry, squirm, and use all kinds of delaying tactics to avoid insulin injections and finger pricks. Sometimes they are angry about being held still or having their play interrupted. Remember how hard it is just to wipe a toddler's nose! They may also be reacting to the fear and anxiety they sense in you. Here are some helpful hints for making injection time go more smoothly:

- Try to take a matter-of-fact approach to the insulin injections and finger pricks.
- Be quick, calm, and reassuring when you carry out these routines.
- Reduce your child's anxious time by getting the dose and/or equipment ready before you involve the child.
- If possible, go where the child is playing to cause less disruption.
- Your child's crying, protests, and other delaying tactics are normal. Remember that, each time you give insulin or do a finger prick, you are helping your child stay healthy.
- Gently hold or restrain your child if he or she struggles.
- Get the needle or finger prick over with quickly. Delaying it only prolongs the agony for everyone.
- Give your child a big hug and kiss after you give the needle, even if he or she didn't cooperate.
- Praise your child for any sign of cooperation.

Can diabetes complicate menstruation?
No, but the hormonal increase prior to or during menstruation can cause blood glucose levels to rise. Some women require more insulin just before or during their periods. This is checked by observing the blood glucose pattern during the menstrual cycle.

Can my teen sleep in on weekends?
Although your diabetes team stresses consistency in the timing of meals and snacks, with a little extra effort and caution your teen can make the adjustments needed to sleep in safely. For example, if he's going to bed at midnight on Saturday night and he wants to sleep in until 10 a.m. Sunday, try this: instead of taking his evening NPH insulin at 10 p.m., take it at midnight, together with a blood glucose check and a little extra snack. (If he's on two injections a day, it's advisable to split the evening one: take the rapid-acting insulin before supper, and take the intermediate-acting at bedtime, along with an added small snack and a blood glucose check.) This will ensure that he doesn't go low during those extra sleep hours.

If your teen is on an insulin pump, sleeping in is much easier. He should stay on his overnight basal rate, and take a bolus with his first meal. The risk of either hypoglycemia or hyperglycemia should be very low.

Can someone with diabetes learn to fly a plane?
People with diabetes have recently challenged the FAA in the United States, and Transport Canada, to reverse a blanket policy banning anyone with diabetes from flying a plane. Now, recreational pilots with diabetes are determined fit for flying based on their individual records of blood glucose control.

I get tired of always being the "bad guy," always saying no when my 12-year-old asks for a treat other than at a meal or snack time—any suggestions?
Some parents handle this situation by reversing the question: "Well, what do you think? Do you think you can have that treat and still keep your blood glucose balanced?" Most often,

the child makes a sensible choice. Sometimes the question leads to creative problem-solving.

My 9-year-old learned to give his own insulin injection at camp last summer and continued to do it regularly for the month after camp. But now he's lost interest and doesn't want to do it anymore. Should we insist that he carry on?
No. It's appropriate for you to take most of the responsibility for injections right now. He'll do it again when he's motivated. If he wants to go on a sleepover he'll have to show you, a little while in advance, that he can safely manage this task.

Another tactic is to pull out a calendar and plan, together, a few days when he's going to give his shot with your supervision. This will maintain his confidence level.

My 6-year-old son has been forgetting to eat his morning snack at school. He's been arriving home quite low at lunch some days. What should I do?
In general, 6-year-olds have no concept of time—and playing in the schoolyard often takes precedence over eating a snack. It's unlikely your son is going to remember to take that snack on his own, and it's reasonable to expect your son's teacher to remind him when it's time. If the snack is interfering with play, consider something fast and easy to eat: for example, a few raisins instead of an apple. Or, if necessary, ask the teacher to give him the snack in class just prior to the recess break.

I have a hard time getting my teen to do a blood glucose check. I know from attending a parents' group meeting that other parents have the same problem. It just takes a few minutes out of their day. Why is it such a problem getting these important checks done?

There are a lot of reasons why teens hate checking their blood glucose levels:

- It's inconvenient and time-consuming—to a teen, losing a few minutes of sleep or party time means a lot.
- Each check is a reminder that they have diabetes and they are not the same as their peers.
- They feel accountable for each blood glucose result—parents frequently demand explanations for high or low readings.
- The results may make them feel guilty—they may know why they're high but be unwilling to do anything about it. It feels better not to check.
- They don't understand the purpose of checking—they don't know how to use the results.
- They feel discouraged by the results, which don't reflect their efforts to manage their diabetes.

It's worthwhile having a discussion with your teen in an attempt to discover what the issues are in his or her particular case.

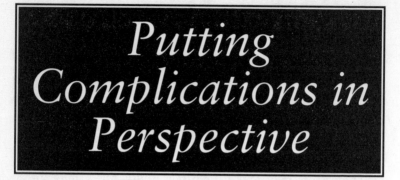

NINE

Putting Complications in Perspective

To 22-year-old Jason, those early days of learning about diabetes are like a long-ago nightmare. They started a little more than 10 years ago, when all he could think of was not missing a hockey game. Now he's thinking about his future. He's almost finished university. He's in love with a girl he met in second year. Will he get a job? Will he get married? Intermingled with thoughts of career and personal relationships are anxieties about his diabetes in the next stage of his life. Will the disease interfere with his long-term plans? If so, what can he do to lessen the risk? His parents have been concerned about these things for years!

After the discovery of insulin, diabetes was no longer immediately life-threatening. Doctors expected that all the problems of the disease would disappear too. Unfortunately this was not the case, and a new set of diabetes-related complications soon began to emerge. Over the last several decades, researchers have learned a great deal about these complications—their symptoms, causes, and treatment—and how to slow their progression. Perhaps most important, researchers are now devising ways to prevent complications altogether.

The best way to prevent complications from diabetes is to maintain the best blood glucose control possible. This is hard work and, because complications are very rare in young people, the threat rarely motivates them. Most young people seldom think about their health twenty years down the road, and children with diabetes are no exception. That's where parents, family members, and health care professionals come in—to provide the foresight and support to help them stay on track toward a healthy future.

The list of potential complications is long and can be quite depressing. But remember, these problems don't affect everyone with diabetes. We also know much more now about how to reduce the risk than even ten years ago.

What Are the Complications of Diabetes?

The physical complications fall into two groups: microvascular (involving small blood vessels) and macrovascular (involving large blood vessels).

Microvascular complications include:
- retinopathy, or eye damage
- nephropathy, or kidney damage
- neuropathy, or nerve damage

Macrovascular complications include:
- cardiovascular disease, or risk of heart attack
- cerebrovascular disease, or risk of stroke
- peripheral vascular disease, or poor circulation to the limbs, which may cause foot problems

While microvascular complications occur only in people with diabetes, macrovascular complications also occur in the general population, but less commonly. Remember, though, that not everyone with diabetes develops these problems.

These complications are virtually unheard of in young children and uncommon during the teenage years. However, diabetes probably starts to have its effect from the time of onset. The impact may be somewhat less before puberty, but early changes seem to accelerate during adolescence. Indeed followup studies from the Diabetes Complications and Control Trial show that early achievement of lower A1C levels is associated with fewer complications later on. This concept, known as "metabolic memory," strongly suggests that efforts to maintain a good blood glucose balance right from the time of diagnosis will contribute to overall long-term health.

Risk Factors for the Development of Diabetes-Related Complications:

- Duration of diabetes: Even the very earliest stages of these complications are rare in those who have had the disease for less than 5 years, and before the onset of puberty. After that, the longer the duration of the diabetes, the more likely it is that complications will arise.
- Inadequate blood glucose control: The Diabetes Control and Complications Trial showed a close relationship between both the onset and the progression of diabetes-related complications, and the degree of long-term blood glucose control. This trial demonstrated clearly that control counts. Independent of any other risk factors, excellent blood glucose control decreases the development of complications. However, that doesn't mean that someone with poor control is 100 percent guaranteed to have complications, nor does it mean that someone with excellent control is guaranteed not to have them.

- Smoking: Many studies show that smokers with diabetes are at much greater risk of developing complications, and having those complications worsen rapidly, than non-smokers. Giving up smoking decreases the risk considerably.
- High blood pressure: People with diabetes who develop high blood pressure (hypertension) are at high risk of complications because of increased pressure on the kidneys, heart, and blood vessels. Lowering the blood pressure with aggressive medical treatment reduces this risk. Regular blood pressure checks are an essential part of diabetes care.
- High blood fats (lipids—cholesterol and triglycerides): People with poor blood glucose control develop high blood fat levels (hyperlipidemia). There are also people who are born with a tendency to develop high blood fat levels. In both cases, these high levels contribute to the risk of complications. Screening for high blood fats is another important part of diabetes care.
- Obesity: People who are markedly overweight are at increased risk for macrovascular complications. Weight control may be a difficult challenge for teens and adults, especially girls.

Screening for Complications in Youth

It is very unusual for children before the onset of puberty, or those who have had diabetes for less than three to five years, to show evidence of long-term complications. Even in teens who have had diabetes for five or ten years, advanced complications are extremely unusual. Nevertheless, once puberty has started and the disease has been present for three to five years, screening for complications and risk factors should begin. If no problems are found, that's reassuring. If the early stages of complications are detected, that allows intervention to prevent them from developing, or at least to slow their progression.

Blood Glucose and Complications— What's the Connection?

Although we know that persistently high blood glucose levels are associated with an increased risk of complications, the connection between the two is still the subject of intense research. It's likely that a number of different mechanisms are involved. For example, glucose sticks to many proteins (as it sticks to hemoglobin, leading to the formation of A1C). Over a long period the attachment of the glucose may change the way some proteins function, and damage the surrounding tissues.

High blood glucose levels also affect the metabolism of many tissues, by altering the rate at which certain molecules are produced or removed. This may lead to a decreased level of molecules that are essential to the way the tissue functions, or the level may be increased enough to damage tissues. Among the tissues affected this way are the nerves and the retina of the eye.

When poor blood glucose control leads to high levels of fat in the blood, that fat may be deposited in the arteries, causing arteriosclerosis (hardening of the arteries)—a major risk factor for macrovascular diseases such as heart attack and stroke. People with diabetes are more likely to develop high blood pressure, which increases the risk of arteriosclerosis and is in itself a risk factor for macrovascular disease.

Here are some blood and urine tests and examinations that your health care team will recommend on a regular basis. More frequent testing will likely be advised if any abnormalities are discovered.

Test/Examination	Frequency
Blood pressure	every 3–6 months
A1C (to assess metabolic control)	every 3–4 months

Test/Examination	*Frequency*
Laboratory blood glucose against your own meter (to check your meter's accuracy)	every 3–6 months
Thyroid function (thyroid stimulating hormone— to detect overfunctioning or underfunctioning of the thyroid)	every 1–2 years
Blood fats (cholesterol including HDL and LDL cholesterol and triglycerides)	3–6 months after diagnosis and, if normal, once again after puberty
tTG—Screening for Celiac Disease	this is a blood test done routinely on children/ teens with diabetes about 3–6 months post diagnosis and every 2 years there after
albumin: creatinine ratio in a random urine sample, or an overnight or 24-hour urine collection for micro-albumin excretion rate (to detect early diabetic nephropathy)	annually after onset of puberty and 3–5 years of diabetes
Eye checkup with ophthal-mologist (to detect early diabetic retinopathy)	annually after onset of puberty and 5 years of diabetes
Dental checkups	every 6 months

Diabetic Retinopathy

Anatomy of the eye

Diabetic retinopathy is damage to the retina, the light-sensitive lining at the back of the eyeball. The condition starts quietly and slowly, with changes seen only on careful examination of the eye by an experienced ophthalmologist or through taking photographs of the retina. In its early and even late stages, retinopathy does not usually interfere with vision. Once vision impairment begins, it suggests that the retinopathy is far advanced.

The earliest changes are called background (non-proliferative) retinopathy, and consist of little swellings of the blood vessels, called microaneurysms, which may start to leak or burst causing leaking (exudates) and bleeding (hemorrhages). Vision is only compromised if the bleeding affects the part of the eye that focuses on the object of vision (the macula), or if that area swells (macular edema). Almost everyone with type 1 diabetes will develop background retinopathy after having the disease for fifteen to twenty years.

Normal retina

Retinopathy

This early stage of retinopathy may progress to proliferative retinopathy, where the eye begins to make new blood vessels to provide better blood flow. These new vessels are fragile and may cause bleeding and scarring in the fluid chamber (vitreous body) in front of the retina. This bleeding is called vitreous hemorrhage, and the scarring can cause detachment of the retina. Proliferative retinopathy and its consequences are a major cause of partial or complete loss of sight. In developed countries, diabetic retinopathy is the most common cause of acquired blindness in adults. However, this does not mean that most people with diabetes will lose their vision.

Researchers have made great strides in repairing vision and reducing the risk of blindness in people with diabetes. Photocoagulation is a laser therapy technique that prevents blindness by destroying abnormal blood vessels, repairing leaking ones, and stopping new ones from forming. This should reduce the risk of blindness by more than 75 to 80 percent. Occasionally, if the retina has bled too much or has become detached, surgery may be required. New medications are also being used to treat diabetic eye disease.

Cataracts

A cataract is a thickening in the lens of the eye. The glucose alcohol sorbitol, a by-product of high blood glucose, is believed to be the cause. Cataracts cause persistent blurring of vision. They are very rarely found in young people with type 1 diabetes, but can develop at any time.

Cataracts can be surgically removed, and the remaining visual impairment corrected with glasses or contact lenses.

Nephropathy

The two kidneys are the body's filtering system. As blood flows through the blood vessels into the kidneys, toxins and waste are removed and transported out of the kidneys, and out of the body, in the urine. The relationship between diabetes and kidney disease is complex. Kidneys may enlarge and become overworked, in a condition called diabetic nephropathy.

Not all people with type 1 diabetes develop nephropathy. It is more likely to occur after puberty, in about one in three people who have had type 1 diabetes for fifteen years or longer. Poor blood glucose control, high blood pressure, and smoking (or chewing) tobacco also increase the risk of kidney failure.

Nephropathy, like retinopathy, develops slowly and quietly, with no symptoms or signs until serious kidney damage has occurred. Symptoms and signs may include:

• higher blood pressure than usual
• puffy ankles due to water retention (edema)
• excessive protein in the urine (proteinuria)
• excessive waste nitrogen levels in the blood (high concentration of creatinine and urea)

Diabetic nephropathy can be detected at a very early stage, before it causes symptoms. This early phase, called incipient nephropathy, is marked by the presence of very small amounts of the protein albumin in the urine. This is called microalbuminuria; it can be detected in a first-morning or random urine specimen. If nephropathy progresses, the amount of protein in the urine will steadily increase to the stage of overt proteinuria. At this stage, protein can be detected by means of a routine protein dipstick in the urine.

Recent research has demonstrated that the onset of diabetic nephropathy can be prevented, or its progression can be significantly slowed, by achieving and maintaining excellent blood glucose control. Further progression can also be prevented or slowed with specific medications called angiotensin converting enzyme or (ACE) inhibitors; or angiotensin II receptor blockers (ARBs).

If nephropathy remains untreated, it will progress to chronic renal (kidney) failure and eventually to end-stage renal failure, which requires dialysis or transplantation if the person is to survive.

Advanced nephropathy is associated with a significant increased risk of macrovascular complications and early death due to diabetes.

Neuropathy

High blood glucoses over the long term can also affect the nerves in many areas of the body. Some slowing of the electrical impulses that travel along the nerves is common in people with diabetes. However, some people go on to develop symptoms and signs of more severe neuropathy. This is extremely rare in children or teens.

Neuropathy commonly affects the nerves to the arms and the legs, and is characterized by:
- tingling in the fingers and toes, extending toward the body
- numbness (loss of feeling) in these areas
- painful burning or freezing sensations, particularly in the feet
- cramping or weakness
- inability to detect hot and cold temperatures

Symptoms of neuropathy can come and go, and are influenced by the level of blood glucose control. Certain prescription medications (such as oxycodone, the antidepressants imipramine or amitriptyline, or the anticonvulsants gabapentin, pregabalin, or clonazepam) may alleviate the pain.

Autonomic neuropathy, which is distinctly unusual in child-hood or adolescence, affects the nerves to internal organs, such as the gastrointestinal system or bladder. When the gastroin-testinal system is affected, there may be problems with the stomach (including vomiting and difficulty moving the food into the intestines, along with bloating, called gastroparesis) or with the intestines (including constipation or, more com-monly, diarrhea). Therapy is difficult, but may include smaller meal sizes and medications to improve intestinal action.

Nerve damage affecting the bladder can lead to urine reten-tion or loss of bladder control. In some cases, men experience sexual dysfunction or impotence. These problems can be improved significantly with better blood glucose control and, if needed, medication.

Foot Problems

The risk of foot problems as a complication of diabetes in chil-dren and adolescents is negligible. As people with diabetes get older, they are more susceptible to infections and slow healing, due to poor circulation and the effects of neuropathy. A person with neuropathy can get a cut on the sole of the foot, or a blister from an ill-fitting shoe, and not even know it. This is espe-cially likely to happen if the injury is the first indicator of neu-ropathy, and the feet are not being examined each day. If the cut remains unnoticed, it can quickly become infected and, in the worst case, lead to gangrene (tissue death). The only recourse then is to amputate the dead tissue.

Although children don't usually experience foot infections, poor healing, or gangrene, it's wise for them to develop good foot care habits so that problems can be avoided as they get older. From an early age, they should be taught how to take good care of their feet, just as they learn how to take good care of their hair, teeth, and other parts of their body. Good foot care means keeping the feet clean and dry—just as anyone would—wearing proper-fitting shoes, cutting toenails straight across rather than rounding them, avoiding ingrown toenails, and getting into the habit of examining the feet for cuts and blisters on a regular basis.

Macrovascular Complications

As people age, so do their large blood vessels. The term for this aging process is arteriosclerosis (often called "hardening of the arteries"). People with type 1 diabetes are susceptible to early aging of their large blood vessels, as are people who smoke, are obese, have persistently high blood fats, or have uncontrolled high blood pressure. Arteriosclerosis can lead to heart attacks or heart failure (cardiovascular disease), strokes (cerebrovascular disease), or foot problems (peripheral vascular disease). As in other complications of diabetes, the risk

---

A Good Health Reminder

The Diabetes Control and Complications Trial proved that the risk of developing microvascular complications can be significantly reduced with careful attention to blood glucose levels. Children can also decrease their risk of complications in adulthood by adopting healthy habits now:

- Eat a healthy diet to maintain normal blood fats and body weight.
- Don't smoke. Every day the list of complications of cigarette smoking gets longer. The effects of smoking are compounded in people with diabetes.
- Keep your blood pressure down. If the body has to work harder than it should to pump blood, the blood vessels and kidneys start to feel the effects. Eye problems may also be aggravated by high blood pressure. You can lower blood pressure by exercising, eating properly (with less salt), and maintaining a healthy weight.
- Get regular exercise, but work it into your plan.

can be reduced by maintaining excellent blood glucose control, keeping blood pressure in check, exercising regularly, eating a healthy diet, and not smoking.

Macrovascular complications are an ominous sign. Fortunately, they are almost unheard of in teens.

Q&A

Is it all right for my 6-year-old daughter with diabetes to go barefoot at the beach?
If you think it is safe for anyone in your family to walk around with bare feet on the beach, then it should be safe for your daughter too. A child with diabetes will have no more trouble healing than other members of the family.

Will our child have difficulty obtaining life insurance policies or any other types of insurance, such as mortgage, car, or home insurance, because of the diabetes?
In the past, insurance companies either were unwilling to provide coverage or else demanded a significantly higher rate for life and other insurance policies for people with diabetes. More recently, with improved care and a better long-term outlook, most insurance companies have become increasingly willing to provide this coverage. It is important that people with diabetes, like anyone else in society, have appropriate insurance. Shop around for the best policies and prices available. Ask advice of your local diabetes association branch or support group, or others you know who have diabetes. Also, don't take no for an answer if your first attempts to get coverage are refused. Keep requesting coverage, and ask your doctor or other health professional to write a letter supporting your application.

Is my child more likely to need glasses because of the diabetes?
Children with diabetes are no more likely than their non-diabetic friends to need glasses for either near- or far-sightedness. Diabetes does not cause permanent problems with vision unless retinopathy has become severe. This is exceptionally rare during childhood and adolescence. Sometimes, rapid changes in blood glucose can cause changes to the lens of the eye— swelling (if the glucose is very high) or contraction (if the glucose is very low). This can cause temporary blurring of vision. Balancing the blood glucose will invariably correct this. Nevertheless, a child who complains of difficulty seeing the chalkboard, or who has to sit close to the television, should have an eye exam to see if glasses are required.

My teenage daughter has diabetes. So far her doctor has not recommended any special eye or kidney tests. Is this okay?
It may be that your doctor has not initiated these checks because your daughter has had diabetes for less than five years. Regular screening should start after the onset of puberty and should also be done for children who have had diabetes longer than five years. If your daughter has had diabetes for that long, don't hesitate to bring up your concerns with your doctor; ask for a referral to an ophthalmologist (eye specialist), and request a urine check for microalbuminuria.

My teenage son has diabetes and his doctor is recommending that he begin regular eye exams with an ophthalmologist instead of the optometrist I see. What is the difference between these two eye doctors?
For people with diabetes, the purpose of regular eye examinations is both to check visual acuity (how well they see) and to examine the interior of the eye for any signs of damage

(retinopathy) that, if left untreated, may interfere with vision. The follow-up and treatment of any retinopathy require the expertise of an ophthalmologist, a physician who specializes in the diagnosis and treatment (both medical and surgical) of eye disorders. An optometrist, who is not a physician, specializes in measuring the refractive power of the lens of the eye and fitting people with glasses or contact lenses. Like the ophthalmologist, the optometrist is expected to put drops in your son's eyes to dilate the pupils in order to do a thorough examination of the back of the eye, using special equipment. Should any retinopathy be detected, your son should be referred to an ophthalmologist, if he is not already seeing one.

Does having diabetes mean that my child is more likely to develop kidney or bladder infections?
Poorly controlled diabetes with very high glucose readings may lead to an increased susceptibility to bladder or vaginal infections. Diabetic nephropathy (kidney damage) does not cause an increased risk of kidney or bladder infection.

Do oral contraceptives increase the risk of diabetes-related complications?
Research shows that women with diabetes but no other risk factors who use the contraceptive pill are not at any greater risk of complications than those who use other forms of contraception. The pills used today have much lower dosages of estrogen (the female hormone) than previously.

Is smoking really bad for people with diabetes?
Yes! There are stacks of research to show that people with diabetes who choose to smoke are at greater risk for developing both microvascular and macrovascular complications. Also,

they are likely to take more time off work or school when they have minor illnesses such as a cold or flu.

I have heard that impotence is a complication of diabetes in men. Is this true?
Some men do experience impotence as a complication of diabetes. This may be the result of nerve damage and circulation problems associated with long-standing diabetes and inadequate blood glucose control. Careful attention to diabetes self-management and blood glucose control is the best way to stay healthy and prevent impotence.

TEN

Setting the Stage for a Healthy Future

On his sixteenth birthday, Paul reached more than one milestone. Soon he would be driving a car, but it was also his tenth year of living with diabetes. Unfortunately, getting Paul to keep diabetes clinic appointments has become increasingly difficult. Either they conflict with an important game or exam, or he complains that, since he feels fine and his blood glucose levels are fine, why should he have to go to the clinic? It's a good thing that Paul's blood glucose levels are so stable. But even when things are going well, there are reasons to stay in touch with the diabetes team. Paul is missing out on the opportunity to learn about changes in diabetes care. For instance, an athlete like Paul would probably benefit from a four-shot-a-day insulin routine, but Paul is behind the times. Also, as Paul gets older he needs to become aware of prevention and screening of complications that may affect him in adulthood. In order to re-establish a baseline and to detect possible changes in eye, kidney, or nerve function, Paul has to see his diabetes team regularly.

As soon as the diagnosis of type 1 diabetes is made, insulin therapy begins and parents and child start an education program to take them through the basics of diabetes management. Once early stabilization and initial education are complete, the major challenge is to maintain health and well-being, both short-term and long-term. This requires regular visits and consultation with the diabetes team and education updates, to prepare the family for new periods in growth and psychosocial development. The continuing focus on health maintenance and health promotion helps motivate and encourage persistent and careful attention to diabetes management. Most of the time, families are able to avoid, or at least deal with, crises before they get out of hand. There are planned educational and support sessions to smooth the transition from one stage of development to the next. In particular, the regular follow-up helps pave the way for the teen to transfer to an adult care diabetes team toward the end of adolescence.

Health Care Follow-Up

Ongoing follow-up is essential. Clinical practice guidelines published by both the Canadian and American Diabetes Associations suggest a minimum of three or four visits per year (every three or four months), and more in the first year of diabetes and for those who need extra support to achieve and maintain good blood glucose control.

Reasons for regular follow-up include:
• assessment of
  – health in general and diabetes in particular
  – growth and development
  – attitudes and behaviors, including school attendance
  – lifestyle issues, e.g., current activities—sleeping in, smoking, alcohol use
  – current and anticipated challenges in living with and coping with diabetes management

- updating and/or clarifying goals and expectations
- anticipatory guidance and joint problem-solving with various members of the team
- support and reassurance
- ongoing education—for parents, children, and teens to learn new skills, concepts, and management measures, and to review important principles and practices
- surveillance for diabetes-related complications, when appropriate
- finding out what is new in research
- having the opportunity to participate in relevant research

The Clinic Visit
Clinic visits are a time to take stock of how well the diabetes is being controlled, how it impacts on the child's and family's lifestyle and how their lifestyle is affecting the diabetes. Visits focus on three areas:
- diabetes-specific issues such as:
  - insulin requirements (frequency, injection sites, timing of injections, types of insulin, dosages)
  - meal planning (including eating attitudes and behavior, particularly in adolescents)
  - results of self-monitoring of blood glucose levels
  - symptoms, frequency, and treatment of hypoglycemia and hyperglycemia
  - physical and other activities that affect blood glucose control
  - sick days
- growth and physical development, including progression of puberty
- psychosocial adjustment, including family stress, school attendance and performance, behavioral issues; and, in the

teen, issues such as smoking, alcohol and drug usage, sexuality and sexual exploration, career planning, and, eventually, transition to adult care

The physical checkup generally includes height and weight measurements to ensure that the child is growing well. The doctor or nurse will also measure blood pressure, feel the thyroid gland (in the neck) and the liver for any enlargement, look at the back of the eye with an ophthalmoscope and inspect insulin injection sites for bumps and lumps.

The regular visits also afford parents and child an opportunity to learn more about diabetes, and become more confident in their ability to make their own routine adjustments. The diabetes team can also help identify any potential psychosocial issues that may affect diabetes management, or vice versa, and begin to deal with them immediately and appropriately.

Since the needs of children with diabetes change as they age, it helps if children and their families can continue to meet the members of their diabetes team from time to time. Many centers offer group meetings where parents can meet other parents and ask questions of experts, while children meet other children with diabetes in a friendly environment. However, group sessions should not replace individual family counseling, which helps to nurture the relationship between the team and the growing child or teen. While these sessions are important for children who are having a hard time achieving blood glucose targets, they are also a valuable support for those with excellent or good control.

The Role of the Family Doctor

The relationship with the diabetes health care team cannot

Thyroid Disease and Diabetes

About one in four or five people with type 1 diabetes will develop alterations in the function of the thyroid gland. While this is associated with diabetes, it is not a complication of long-standing or poorly controlled diabetes. The thyroid is found in the lower part of the front of the neck, and is responsible for production of the thyroid hormones (thyroxine or T4 and tri-iodothyronine or T3), which are important regulators of growth and metabolism.

The thyroid may be the target of an autoimmune response similar to the one that affects the beta cells in the pancreas and causes diabetes. This thyroid damage is known as Hashimoto's thyroiditis and may cause underactivity of the thyroid gland (hypothyroidism). If the thyroid starts to become underactive, the body's metabolism slows. This may reveal itself in slower growth, weight gain, tiredness or sluggishness, dry skin and hair, constipation and, in women, menstrual irregularities.

Regular checks of thyroid function allow detection of underactivity before symptoms become evident. Checks involve measuring the level of the hormone TSH, or thyroid stimulating hormone, made in the pituitary gland, in the brain. As the thyroid gland starts to fail, the pituitary gland makes more TSH in an attempt to bolster thyroid function. An elevated TSH level is therefore the best indicator of impending thyroid failure. If thyroid underactivity is detected, it can be treated with levothyroxine, a synthetic form of thyroid hormone, in the form of a small pill.

In rare instances the thyroid gland becomes overactive. Symptoms of hyperthyroidism (Graves' disease) may include weight loss with increased appetite, mood swings, shakiness and sweating, diarrhea, and prominence of the eyes. This can be treated with thyroid-suppressing medications.

and should not replace the role of the family doctor or pediatrician in attending to the child's general health. Routine immunization, managing infections, and annual physicals should continue outside the diabetes team. Good communication is essential. Parents and diabetes specialists should keep the family doctor informed about the child's diabetes management plan. Likewise, the family doctor will communicate any concerns to the rest of the diabetes team.

Getting the Most out of the Visit with Your Health Care Team
Over the years the family dealing with diabetes will become
quite familiar with the health care system. Some people take
a while to become comfortable working with health care professionals, but remember that the diabetes team is there for
the family. Here are some tips on how to get the most from
your health care team.

Before the visit
- write out questions and concerns so you won't forget things
- write down any recent symptoms
- keep self-monitoring records current
- know and follow the standards of care
- know what the previous A1C was
- rehearse the main points you want to cover

During the visit
- remember to bring the blood glucose logbook and the
  glucose meter
- request time to ask questions
- write down the answers
- repeat answers back to the health care provider for clarity
- make a specific plan of action for any changes to the diabetes routine
- make an appointment for the next visit
- ask if thyroid and blood fat tests should be done. If the child
  has reached puberty and has had diabetes for three to five
  years, ask if it is time to begin screening for eye and kidney
  changes

After the visit
- list the recommendations given

- decide to implement them
- tell the rest of the family
- encourage the child to keep a diary to help keep track of the routine
- phone to get the A1C result from the previous visit if it was not available before you left the clinic
- phone to get results from any other screening tests

Moving from Pediatric to Adult Health Care

Although children with diabetes have special needs and benefit from care given by health care providers experienced in childhood diabetes, there comes a time when the teenager needs to link up with a team experienced in the care of adults.

This transition can be quite emotional and stressful for all. Moving on to a new health care setting is like graduating from high school to college. Over a short period of time, the teenager shifts from being the biggest, oldest, and wisest person to being a young, inexperienced rookie in a larger and different environment. Some find the experience exciting, while others prefer the security of the old setting. Expectations for self-management and control differ between pediatric and adult care. In the adult system, young adults are often seen as taking complete responsibility for themselves.

As teens enter the adult system, many are surprised by the demands placed on them. If they are not already doing so, they may be expected to practice more intensive management of their diabetes, aiming for tighter blood glucose control through more frequent injections and glucose monitoring. There will be changes in meal plans, as they are no longer growing. Some find they are not as physically active as they used to be, and have to compensate for that with a more structured exercise regimen. As their risk of complications increases with age, they may have to monitor blood pressure and see an eye doctor more frequently. Routine foot care will be emphasized, to prevent infections and identify signs of nerve damage. These demands can be overwhelming and the newly graduated teenager can feel incapable of meeting them. Some young adults are tempted to drop out of care altogether. The support of family and friends throughout the transition phase is vital to ensure that the young adult continues with the care needed to manage his or her diabetes.

Ideally, the change to adult care should come when the teenager is confident and responsible enough to move forward. Unfortunately, hospital or clinic policy usually dictates a transition between the ages of 16 and 20. Parents and teens should be aware of this well ahead of time in order to prepare.

Parents can help teens make a successful transfer by encouraging them to take an active part in their diabetes care throughout childhood and adolescence. When parents encourage their children to problem-solve and make choices about adjusting insulin doses, for example, they set the foundation for the self-management behaviors essential in adulthood. Teenagers also need private time with all members of the diabetes team, as this promotes independence and responsibility. Before being discharged from the pediatric center, teens should have the opportunity to explore various options for continuing their diabetes health care, and a referral should be made to the adult team. It is also helpful for a teen leaving the pediatric center to take part in either an individual or a group program that stresses the need for ongoing excellent blood glucose control, surveillance for complications, and changing expectations.

Q&A

Our daughter has diabetes. Are there any special precautions we should take when we go on our summer holiday?

Your daughter's diabetes should not discourage you from traveling—even abroad. Unfortunately, you can't take a vacation from her diabetes. But careful planning will ensure a safe and enjoyable holiday. Here are some tips:

- Take enough insulin and other supplies to last for the entire trip, and some to spare. Keep the extra in a separate location from the main supply, in case one of your bags is lost or stolen.
- Take a letter (from a member of your diabetes team) explaining the need to carry sharps, juice boxes, etc., through security.
- If you're boarding a plane, make sure all your supplies are in your carry-on baggage.
- Wherever you go, always carry some food, together with a good supply of fast-acting glucose to treat insulin reactions.
- Plan to monitor blood glucose at least four or more times a day—specifically, before meals and at bedtime. The routine will be different than it is at home, and you'll need to know how her blood glucose is affected so you can make safe adjustments.
- For active holidays, you may need to reduce your daughter's insulin. Speak with members of your diabetes team.
- Make sure your daughter wears some form of diabetes identification, such as a medical-alert bracelet.
- Be prepared for emergencies. Take the glucagon kit with you, so you can respond to severe low blood glucose if necessary. And take your sick-day guidelines and your ketone testing strips with you.
- Don't forget to take the phone numbers of key members of

your diabetes team. They may also be able to provide you with the names of experts in your holiday location.

How do I deal with a time-zone change?

There is no magic formula to help you figure out how to adjust insulin for a time-zone change—every situation and individual is different. Know the time action of your insulins inside out, and gather all the information you can about your flight—time change and available food (you'll bring along extra, of course). Then sit down with your doctor or nurse to figure out a plan. Those who are on insulin pump therapy or an MDI (multiple daily insulin) routine with long- and rapid-acting insulin with food will find it much easier to deal with time zone changes.

Is it hard to get travel insurance?

As with life and other forms of insurance, it can be more difficult for people with diabetes to obtain travel insurance. The Canadian Diabetes Association offers travel insurance to members. Contact your nearest branch or go online for more information.

My son wants to go on a ten-day camping trip into the wilderness. He will be out of contact with civilization for most of the time. Should I let him go?

This is a decision for you and your son to make. Before letting him go, you should feel comfortable that he and his friends understand the issues involved in being out in the wilderness. Your son should have demonstrated good judgment and a high level of responsibility in diabetes care, and should be committed to doing more, rather than less, blood glucose testing on the trip. You should make every effort to ensure that there is some method of communication with "civilization" if at all possible.

After my daughter "graduates" from the diabetes clinic at the hospital, isn't it okay for her to be seen by her family doctor only?

It's still important for your daughter to have access to all members of the diabetes health care team (doctor, nurse, dietitian, social worker), even after she leaves the children's clinic. There are obstacles to negotiate at each age and stage of development, such as moving away to college or university, living on her own, changes in exercise or activity patterns, frequent trips away from home on business—the list goes on and on. These are best dealt with by health care professionals experienced in diabetes care. If your family doctor is one of these, then he or she may well meet your daughter's needs.

I've heard that people with diabetes are more susceptible to something called celiac disease. Is this true? And what is celiac disease?

Celiac disease is an autoimmune disorder, like diabetes or thyroid disease, where the body develops a sensitivity to gluten, the major protein in wheat, barley, and rye. Celiac disease affects the ability of the small intestines to absorb food. Some people have minimal symptoms, but others experience abdominal pain and bloating, poor growth or weight gain, and loose, foul-smelling stools.

People with type 1 diabetes do have a greater chance of developing celiac disease—about one chance in twenty to thirty—and the disease can interfere with diabetes control.

If someone else in your family has the disease, be sure to tell the diabetes team. Many diabetes teams do screening tests for celiac disease on a regular basis.

Diagnosis is made by a blood test and confirmed by a biopsy of the intestine. Treatment consists of avoiding gluten-containing products.

ELEVEN

The Future of Diabetes

Samantha is an inquisitive, freckle-faced girl who has had diabetes for six years. Now 13, she recently began giving her own injections. For the past three years she has been doing her blood glucose checks and she is comfortable taking some glucose tablets when she feels low at her skating lesson. When she first developed diabetes Samantha didn't want to tell anybody, but within six months she gave her first "talk" to her grade two classmates about what it was like to have diabetes. Last year, she won an essay contest with her biography of Frederick Banting.

Samantha likes to surf the Web and often looks for innovations in diabetes. She hopes that one day she won't have to take insulin via injection any longer. At each clinic visit she has a long list of questions for her doctor about new research in diabetes.

Since the discovery of insulin, important advances in the understanding of the cause, course, and treatment of both type 1 and type 2 diabetes have continued to be made. But only some of these advances have led to significant changes in the lives of those with the disease. Media reports of "breakthroughs" often offer unrealistic hope to children with diabetes and their parents: hope that their lives are to be dramatically changed in the very near future. Reality is often different; advances in biomedical research usually take many years to proceed through the appropriate stages of testing, first in test-tubes, then in animals, and finally in people. Sometimes, research that at first seems successful doesn't work out in the long run. While it's disappointing that these experiments don't always lead to new treatment approaches, they often advance our understanding of diabetes in substantial ways. So read the newspaper or watch the news with a critical eye, and get as much information as you can from health care professionals, diabetes journals, and other sources before forming an opinion.

Some people with diabetes (as well as those with other conditions) are quite cynical, believing that the research and medical communities have the ability to cure their disease, but that there is too much profit to be made from not doing so. Nothing could be further from the truth. Both type 1 and type 2 diabetes pose a massive public health burden. It has been suggested that more than 10 percent of all health care expenditures are related in some way to diabetes. A cure is in everyone's best interests. However, a cure may be more elusive than the optimists or the media would have us believe.

Researching the Cause and Possible Cure

In Chapter One we talked about diabetes being an autoimmune disorder, caused when a genetic predisposition or susceptibility is triggered by an environmental stimulus. Over the past twenty years there have been enormous advances in our understanding of the genetic aspects of type 1 diabetes, although pieces of the puzzle remain to be found.

The Genetic Link

There are a number of genes involved in making a person susceptible to type 1 diabetes; the most important appears to lie in the HLA (histocompatibility locus antigen or "tissue typing") region of chromosome six. This region contains genes that control the body's immune responses—for example, how we deal with foreign materials such as viruses, bacteria, and toxins. In those susceptible to diabetes, these genes appear to be somewhat impaired. Contained in this region of chromosome six are different genes that determine different levels of susceptibility, and some actually confer resistance to diabetes! Could this resistance be harnessed and turned into a gene therapy that could alter these impaired genes and protect against diabetes? This is an important research question, but the answer is still a long way off.

The Environmental Link

In the hunt for environmental triggers that may "wake up" a genetic predisposition to diabetes, there has been extensive research focusing on viruses, food products—such as exposure to cow's milk protein early in life—and environmental toxins. This research has not yielded consistent results, nor has it identified a single trigger for the development of diabetes. Researchers hope to identify a viral or other infectious agent responsible for causing the pancreatic damage, so they can work on developing a vaccine against it. This could conceivably prevent diabetes. Avoiding certain toxins could have a similar effect. There are studies in progress that test these hypotheses in both animals and humans.

Preventing the Immunological Response

Once the genes and environment align themselves in a way that starts the progression toward diabetes, a series of known events occur that are now quite well understood and are being studied in greater detail. The immune system and environmental abnormalities lead to an inflammatory response (insulitis) in the islet cells where insulin is made. Antibodies to some of the proteins in the islets appear in the blood. Detecting these antibodies allows us to determine who may be at high risk for developing diabetes.

Most of the studies have been and are being performed on close relatives (parents, children, and siblings) of people with diabetes, because—as you'd expect in any disorder with a genetic link—the risk to family members is much higher than in the general population.

The problem is that diabetes in family members accounts for only 5 to 10 percent of all new cases of type 1 diabetes. Studies in the general population have been much more difficult to perform, and may not be as useful for predictions as those in close relatives.

Studies in animals, such as certain breeds of mice and rats that spontaneously develop an autoimmune type of diabetes very similar to that seen in people, have shown that diabetes can be prevented by exposure to a number of medications that dampen the immunological response. These include some medications with serious side-effects, such as those used to prevent rejection of transplanted organs, as well as much safer agents, such as the vitamin B3 derivative nicotinamide and the hormone insulin. Present studies in Canada, the United States, and Europe are evaluating the possibility of preventing diabetes in high-risk groups by giving these types of medications.

Preventing the Progression of Diabetes
For those who already have diabetes, two different lines of

research are looking at ways to reverse the condition: immune interventions at diagnosis to stop further damage to the pancreas and maintain the "honeymoon period"; and transplanting the pancreas, or at least the islet cells, to reverse the condition once it is fully established. So far interventions at diagnosis have been either unsuccessful or minimally successful and there are currently no treatments approved for routine use.

Whole-Pancreas Transplants

The first whole-pancreas transplants were attempted in the 1960s, and transplants continue to be performed in many centers around the world. The problem with this operation is that the transplanted pancreas is subject to rejection. Recipients must therefore receive high doses of anti-rejection medications, which can have troublesome and significant side-effects, including development of cancer and type 2 diabetes. For people who need a kidney transplant for advanced diabetes-related kidney complications and who will require the use of anti-rejection drugs anyway, transplanting the pancreas at the same time makes good sense. For those well controlled on insulin, with no evidence of kidney complications, transplantation is a less obvious choice. Virtually no transplants have been performed in young people with diabetes.

Islet-Cell Transplants

Enormous efforts have been made not only to perfect pancreatic transplantation, but also to isolate the islets and transplant them without the non-insulin-producing parts of the pancreas. Recent advances in islet-transplantation technology have improved the outlook for this procedure, but extensive testing is still required before it becomes more commonplace. People who receive transplanted islet cells require immunosuppressive drugs thereafter, to prevent rejection of the transplanted cells. Even if the technical and rejection problems can be remedied, it is expected that two to three organ donors' pancreases will be needed for each islet transplant recipient. This is a major stumbling block to islet-cell transplants becoming a realistic solution to type 1 diabetes.

Creating New Islet Cells

The next phase of research involves genetic engineering, in which either animal or non-islet cells are genetically changed to become functioning islet cells. The enormous complexity of islet cell function is being unravelled steadily. This is helping researchers target the genes that must function to make the cells produce and secrete insulin in response to changes in blood glucose levels.

Making Treatment Easier

Although the basic treatment of type 1 diabetes has changed little over the past seventy-five years in terms of the need for insulin injections, major advances have been made in a number of areas:

- the variety and purity of insulin preparations, and methods for delivering insulin under the skin, such as insulin pens and pumps
- new and ever-improving methods for monitoring blood glucose and other measures of blood glucose control, such as the hemoglobin A1C test
- the team approach and other approaches to lifestyle management to help prevent psychosocial and long-term physical side-effects.

Insulin

For many years, the only insulins available were relatively impure preparations of beef and pork insulin. While these were effective in controlling blood glucose levels, they were sometimes associated with side-effects. Over the past thirty years, we have progressed through the development of highly purified pork insulin, to the availability of genetically engineered human insulins, to the recent production of insulin analogs, which are insulins that have been chemically or genetically altered to change their time course of action. The vast majority of people with newly diagnosed type 1 diabetes receive treatment with human insulin, and, for many, a rapid-acting insulin analog is part of their management. There are further new insulin analogs in various stages of development. Some will be alternatives to rapid-acting insulin; others will try to provide the ideal longer-acting basal insulin to which rapid-acting insulin is added at mealtime. Insulin glargine (Lantus) and insulin detemir (Levemir) are the two apparently peakless, long-acting insulin analogs that are already available in many countries.

Insulin Delivery Systems

Better syringes, finer needles, and insulin pens have made insulin injections less painful and more convenient. Smaller and more reliable insulin infusion pumps have also been developed. Pumps don't eliminate the need for a needle or for careful attention to blood glucose control, but they do allow for flexibility in the timing of meals without compromising safety or control. Pumps are meeting with increasing enthusiasm among children and teens.

Scientists also continue to work on other methods to administer insulin—for example, by inhalation through the mouth or nose, or through a patch on the skin. This is a highly fertile area of research, in which advances can be expected in the years to come.

Blood Glucose Monitoring

In the late 1970s, urine glucose testing began to be replaced by blood glucose monitoring, a major advance in diabetes management. Over the next twenty years there were significant improvements in monitoring systems, with the development of smaller, more reliable, user-friendly meters with enhanced memory systems, as well as easier-to-use finger-pricking devices.

There have been two major research thrusts in the field of glucose monitoring: continuous glucose monitoring systems, and non-invasive blood glucose testing devices. These devices would accomplish two things: they would eliminate the need to repeatedly prick the fingers to check blood glucose, and they'd provide the impetus to develop an implantable artificial pancreas, which would detect blood glucose highs or lows, then trigger an insulin pump to infuse the right amount of insulin at the right time. To date, research in this area has been plentiful but a functioning device remains elusive.

Where Do We Go from Here?

Around the world, many researchers remain focused on questions to do with the causes, course, and complications of both type 1 and type 2 diabetes. They continue to make steady progress, but for many people the pace is too slow. It is clear that there is an ever-increasing need for funding to support research and treatment programs.

Children with diabetes, their families and health care providers, and government and non-governmental organizations that fund diabetes care and research must focus on the challenge at hand: to provide the best available care for people with the disease. It is easy to become disillusioned. Those receiving insulin injections will always hope that a major advance is just around the corner. We need, however, to balance this hope against the reality of where we are in biomedical research, and how much we are likely to advance in the next few years. Following the steps to maintain excellent physical and emotional health now is of critical importance. That way, when something better comes along in way of a treatment or cure, your children will be well positioned to benefit from them.

Q&A

I keep reading about ancient cures for diabetes and alternative non-drug remedies. How do I know what to believe?
Children with type 1 diabetes require insulin, which is not a drug. And unfortunately there is no therapy, alternative or otherwise, that eliminates that need. Some people with diabetes find certain nutritional supplements make them feel better. These are probably not harmful, but shouldn't be thought of as part of the diabetes routine. Check with your doctor before taking them.

How can I make sure that I hear about the latest important research in diabetes?
Look to your diabetes team to keep you informed about research that will make a difference to you or your child. It is their responsibility to stay up to date on current treatments and significant advances.

Join the Canadian or American Diabetes Association, and the Juvenile Diabetes Research Foundation. Membership in all organizations includes a subscription to their publications, which always include the latest research. You may also find useful information on the Internet; see Further Resources, at the end of this book.

We are a family of five. One of our children has diabetes. How can the rest of us find out if we are at high risk for developing diabetes, and be part of a prevention study?
The best way to learn about important clinical research and how you can be involved is to talk to members of your diabetes team. If your child is not receiving ongoing care from a pediatric diabetes team and your doctor is unaware of research opportunities that may interest you, you may want to request referral to a children's center.

Every week I read a story in the paper about some new treatment for diabetes being just around the corner. Yet I have had diabetes for twenty-five years and my child has had it for six years, and we're still having insulin injections, doing more testing, and worrying about control. Why do the media report premature research findings?
It's true that a "cure" always seems to be around the corner. There are many reasons why stories often promise more than they deliver. Sometimes, the media misinterpret or sensationalize the information they receive from medical meetings or medical journals. Other times, the researchers themselves give an overly optimistic view of when their research will bear fruit and change the face of diabetes care. Still other times, research that looks promising in its early stages turns out to be not so exciting as the studies continue. Unexpected problems may emerge as treatments are studied over the long haul; initially promising results may not hold up. Read media reports carefully, and ask your health care team or diabetes association about them.

Table of Insulin Types

Type	Made by	Appearance	Timing of Action (in hours)		
			Onset	Peak	Duration
Rapid-acting					
Humalog (lispro)	Eli Lilly	clear	5–10 (min.)	1/2–2	3–4
NovoRapid/NovoLog (aspart)	Novo Nordisk	clear	5–10 (min.)	1/2–2	3–4
*Apidra (glulisine)	sanofi-aventis	clear	5–10 (min.)	1/2–2	3–4
*Not yet licensed in Canada for kids aged four years and up, approval is expected in 2010/11, check with your doctor.					
Short-Acting					
Humulin R (regular)	Eli Lilly	clear	1/2–1	2–5	6–8
Novolin Toronto R	Novo Nordisk	clear	1/2–1	2–5	6–8
Intermediate-Acting					
Humulin N (NPH)	Eli Lilly	cloudy	1–21/2	6–15	18–24
Novolin N (NPH)	Novo Nordisk	cloudy	1–21/2	6–15	18–24
Long-Acting					
Lantus (glargine)	sanofi-aventis	clear	2–4	no peak	24–36
Levemir (detemir)	Novo Nordisk	clear	2–4	almost peakless	18–24
Mixtures *(numbers show percentage of regular/NPH)*					
Humulin	Eli Lilly	30/70, Humalog Mix25, Humalog Mix50			
Novolin	Novo Nordisk	30/70, 40/60, 50/50, NovoMix 30			

Glossary

Albuminuria: presence of protein in the urine. In small amounts, called microalbuminuria, this signals early diabetic nephropathy. Larger amounts, called overt proteinuria or macroproteinuria, suggest advanced nephropathy.

Angiotensin converting enzyme (ACE) inhibitors: medications used to protect the kidney once early nephropathy or high blood pressure has been detected.

Antibodies: proteins produced by the immune system to neutralize foreign proteins (i.e., infectious agents).

Autoimmune disorder: a disease in which the body's immune system mistakenly attacks the body's own tissues.

Type 1 diabetes is the result of an autoimmune disorder.

Basal insulin: the background insulin required to manage blood glucose during sleep and during periods of fasting throughout the day.

Bolus insulin: short- or rapid-acting insulin that is given with carbohydrate-containing meals and snacks or used to correct blood glucose levels that are higher than target.

Beta cells: cells in the pancreas that produce insulin.

Carbohydrate: A major source of energy for the body (sugar and starches).

Correction factor: refers to the units of insulin required to correct an out-of-target blood glucose so that it returns to the desired range.

Diabetic ketoacidosis (DKA): severe dehydration and acidosis that develop when blood glucose is very high and not enough insulin is available to prevent excessive breakdown of fat.

Diabetologist: physician specializing in the care of people with diabetes.

DKA: see Diabetic ketoacidosis.

Endocrinologist: physician specializing in the diagnosis and treatment of diabetes and other disorders involving the endocrine (glandular) system.

Glucagon: hormone produced in the pancreas that increases blood glucose by stimulating the liver to release its glucose stores.

Glucose: the form of glucose required by the cells of the body to supply energy. Sometimes used interchangeably with "sugar."

Glycogen: substance made up of glucose that is stored in the liver and muscles. When cells require glucose for energy, glycogen is changed back into glucose and released into the blood.

Gram: unit of weight in the metric system. There are approximately 30 grams in 1 ounce.

Hemoglobin A1C: blood test used to measure long-term glucose control. Glucose attaches to the hemoglobin in red blood cells in proportion to the average blood glucose level over the lifespan of the red cell (about three months). Measuring A1C levels every three months is the best way to track long-term glucose control.

HLA (histocompatibility locus antigens): "tissue-typing" genes on chromosome six that can control the body's immune response and provide information on someone's risk of developing diabetes.

Immune system: a complex system that defends the body against viruses, bacteria, and other invaders. Sometimes the system malfunctions; see Autoimmune disorder.

Insulin: hormone produced in the pancreas that is essential for normal metabolism of glucose.

Insulin analog: insulin biologically altered to change its onset, peak, and duration of action.

Insulin to carbohydrate ratio: the amount of carbohydrate, measured in grams that 1 unit of insulin metabolizes. This ratio varies from one person to the next and may even vary throughout the day for any one person.

Insulin receptors: areas of body cells to which insulin attaches to allow glucose to enter the cells.

Islet cell antibodies: antibodies to proteins in the pancreas, often found at the time of diagnosis (or even before diagnosis) of diabetes. Used to detect those at risk of diabetes.

Ketoacidosis: see Diabetic ketoacidosis.

Kussmaul breathing: deep, sighing breathing that occurs in diabetic ketoacidosis.

Lipids: fats.

Macrovascular complications: diabetes-related complications that affect the large blood vessels, causing heart attacks, strokes, and poor circulation to the extremities, most commonly the feet.

Macula: area near the center of the eye's retina, responsible for precise vision.

Microalbuminuria: see Albuminuria.

Microvascular complications: diabetes-related complications that affect the small blood vessels, such as nephropathy, neuropathy, and retinopathy.

Nephropathy: kidney damage that may occur as a result of diabetes.

Neuropathy: nerve damage that may occur as a result of diabetes.

Ophthalmologist: physician who specializes in the diagnosis and treatment of diseases of the eye.

Overt proteinuria: see Albuminuria.

Pancreas: organ in the abdomen, behind the stomach, that produces both digestive juices and hormones such as insulin and glucagon.

Retina: center part of the back lining of the eye, which senses light. Its many small blood vessels may become damaged when someone has diabetes for a long time.

Retinopathy: eye damage that may occur as a result of diabetes.

Target range: range of blood glucose within which most results of blood glucose testing should fall.

Thyroid: gland in the lower neck that makes thyroid hormones.

Type 1 diabetes: a form of diabetes that usually begins in childhood and requires treatment with insulin.

Type 2 diabetes: a form of diabetes that usually develops as people age, and can usually be managed through changes in diet and lifestyle.

Further Resources

Organizations

U.S.

The American Diabetes
  Association
1701 North Beauregard Street
Alexandria, VA 22311
Toll-free: 1-800-DIABETES
(1-800-342-2383)
Web: www.diabetes.org
E-mail: AskADA
  @diabetes.org

The Juvenile Diabetes
  Research Foundation
  International
120 Wall Street, 19th Floor
New York, NY 10005-4001
Phone: 212-785-9595
Toll-free: 1-800-533-2873
Web: www.jdrf.org
E-mail: info@jdrf.org

Canada

The Canadian Diabetes
  Association
1400–522 University Avenue
Toronto, ON M5G 2R5
Toll-free: 1-800-BANTING
(1-800-226-8464)
Web: www.diabetes.ca
E-mail: info@diabetes.ca

The Juvenile Diabetes Research
  Foundation Canada
7100 Woodbine Avenue,
Suite 311
Markham, ON L3R 5J2
905-944-8700
Fax: 905-944-0800
Toll-free: 1-877-287-3533
Web: www.jdrf.ca
E-mail: general@jdrf.ca

Websites

British Columbia's Children's Hospital
endodiab.bcchildrens.ca

Canadian group, informal experiential learning, events, blogs:
www.connectedinmotion.ca

Children with Diabetes
www.childrenwithdiabetes.org

Diabetes Exercise and Sports Association (DESA)
www.diabetes-exercise.org/resources.

Hospital for Sick Children, Toronto
www.aboutkidshealth.ca/diabetes

Books

American Diabetes Association. *Reflections on Diabetes: 39 Inspirational, Real-life Stories on Living with Diabetes.* Alexandria, VA: American Diabetes Association, 1996.

Betschart, Jean. *It's Time to Learn about Diabetes: A Workbook on Diabetes for Children.* Minneapolis: Chronimed, 1991.

Betschart, Jean, and Susan Tomm. *In Control: A Guide for Teens with Diabetes.* Minneapolis: Chronimed, 1995.

Betschart-Roemer, Jean. *Diabetes Care for Babies, Toddlers, and Preschoolers: A Reassuring Guide.* Minneapolis: Chronimed, 1999.

Brackenridge, Betty. *Draw Wide the Circle of Love.* Learning Prescriptions, 2008.

Brackenridge, Betty, and R. Rubin. *Sweet Kids: How to Balance Control and Good Nutrition with Family Peace.* Atlanta: American Diabetes Association, 1996.

Chase, Peter. *Understanding Diabetes. A handbook for people who are living with diabetes*. 11th edition. Denver: Paros Press, 2006.

Estridge, Bonnie, and Jo Davies. *Diabetes and Your Teenager*. London: Thursons, with the British Diabetes Association, 1996.

Hanas, Ragnar. *Type 1 Diabetes in Children, Adolescents and Young Adults*. London: Class Publishing, 2009.

Heegaard, Marge, and Chris Ternand. *When a Family Gets Diabetes*. Minneapolis: DCI, 1990.

Hollerorth, Hugo J., and Debra Kaplan, with Anna Maria Bertorelli and Joslin Diabetes Center. *Everyone Likes to Eat: How Children Can Eat Most of the Foods They Enjoy and Still Take Care of Their Diabetes*. Minneapolis: Chronimed, 1993.

Kaufman, Miriam. *Easy for You to Say. Q and As For Teens Living With Chronic Illness or Disabilities*. Toronto: Firefly Books, 2005.

Kaufman, Miriam. *Mothering Teens: Understanding the Adolescent Years*. Toronto: Key Porter, 1997.

Lawlor, M., L. Laffel, B. Anderson, and A. Bertorelli. *Caring for Young Children Living with Diabetes—Parent Manual*. Boston: Joslin Diabetes Center, 2001.

Loring, Gloria. *Parenting a Child with Diabetes: A Practical, Empathetic Guide to Help You and Your Child Live with Diabetes*. Los Angeles: Howell House, 1999.

Nasmyth Loy, Spike and Bo Nasmyth Loy. *487 Really Cool Tips for Kids with Diabetes*. American Diabetes Association, 2004.

Polonsky, William. *Diabetes Burnout: What To Do When You Can't Take It Anymore*. Alexandria, VA: American Diabetes Association, 2000.

Scjeomer, Barry. *Think Like a Pancreas: A practical guide to managing diabetes with insulin*. New York: Marlowe and Company, 2004.

Wysocki, Tim. *The Ten Keys to Helping Your Child Grow Up with Diabetes*. Alexandria, VA: American Diabetes Association, 1997.

Zosel, Renea Jo. *Diabetes: An Emotional Journey*. Covington, WA: Zay Publishing, 2003.

Cookbooks

Bartley, Collen. *Canada's Best Cookbook for Kids with Diabetes*. Toronto: Robert Rose, 2005.

Holzmeister, Lea Ann. *The Diabetes Carbohydrate & Fat Gram Guide*, Third Edition. Alexandria, VA: American Diabetes Association and the American Dietetic Association, 2005.

McClendon, Marie, and Cristy Shauck. *The Healthy Lunchbox: How to Plan, Prepare & Pack Stress-Free Meals Kids Will Love*. Alexandria, VA: Small Steps Press, 2005.

Warshaw, Hope S. *Guide to Healthy Fast-Food Eating*. Alexandria, VA: American Diabetes Association, 2006.

Yasui, Doreen, and Doreen Hatton. *Food and Diabetes— For Kids, Teens, Families and Caregivers*. Vancouver: Children's and Women's Health Centre of British Columbia, 2002.

Multimedia
Living with Diabetes: Tips for Teachers, produced by Max-ishare Productions, Milwaukee, WI, in association with the Wisconsin Connection for Children, Hospital of Wisconsin. 1-414-266-3428

Supporting Students with Type 1 Diabetes in the Classroom. A 20 minute DVD and Booklet. Trillium Paediatric Diabetes Centre, Trillium Health Centre, 100 Queensway West, Mississauga, Ontario, Canada, L5B 1B8 Fax: 905-804-7741

Other Resources
Countdown Canada. Published quarterly by the Juvenile Diabetes Research Foundation Canada. More information at www.jdrf.ca.

Diabetes Dialogue. Published quarterly by the Canadian Diabetes Association. More information at www.diabetes.ca/about-diabetes/literature/diabetes-dialogue.

Diabetes Forecast. Published monthly by the American Diabetes Association. More information at www.diabetes.org.

Diabetes Self-Management. Published bi-monthly by R.A. Rappaport Publishing, New York, NY. 1-800-234-0923. Also available at www.diabetesselfmanagement.com

Index

In this index, page numbers in italic indicate that the information is in a figure or table.

For definitions, see the Glossary on pages 229–32.

jet injectors, 55
juvenile diabetes *see* type 1
    diabetes
Juvenile Diabetes Research
    Foundation, 226

ketoacidosis *see* diabetic
    ketoacidosis
ketone meters, 96
ketones
    during illness, *135*
    harmful body products,
        11, 15–16
ketone tests, *95–96*
kidney failure, 200
kidneys
    nephropathy, 199–200
    normal functioning,
        198–99

labels on foods, 74
lancing devices, 93, *93*
Langerhans, Paul, 3, 36
Lantus insulin, *38*, 224, *228*
legumes, 70, 84
Levemir insulin, *38*, 224, *228*

MacLeod, J.J.R., 37
macrovascular complications,
    202–3
Maturity Onset Diabetes in the
    Young, 19
meals *see* diet
meat, 70
medical-alert bracelets, 140, 215
menstruation, 186
microalbuminuria, 195, 199
Minkowski, Oscar, 36

needles
    fear/dislike of, 40, 57–58
    lengths and thicknesses,
        41, 41
    using, 40, 43–45, 224
nephropathy, 198–200, 205
neuropathy, 200–201
nicotinamide, 221
non-insulin-dependent diabetes
    see type 2 diabetes
Novolin insulin, *228*
Novo Nordisk, 39
NovoRapid insulin, *38*, *228*
NPH insulin, *38*, *228*
Nutrition Facts panels on foods,
    74
nuts, 70

obesity, 5–6, 18–19, 193, 202
oils, 70–71

pancreas
    in diabetes, 4, 20–21
    normal functioning, 3, 10,
        11, 14, 20–21
    research, 36, 222
    transplant, 222
peanut butter, 70
pens and cartridges, 44–45, 58,
    224
piloting, 187
pregnancy, 6–7
preschoolers *see* toddlers
protein, 70
proteinuria, 199
pumps
    adjustments for sick days,
        136–39
    candidates for, 141–42